get ready for Curvy Chic, the ultimate fashion coloring book for women who love their bodies! Unleash your creativity and show off your style. This book is all about celebrating your curves and your personality. So grab your coloring tools and let's have some fun!

- Wonder Word Works

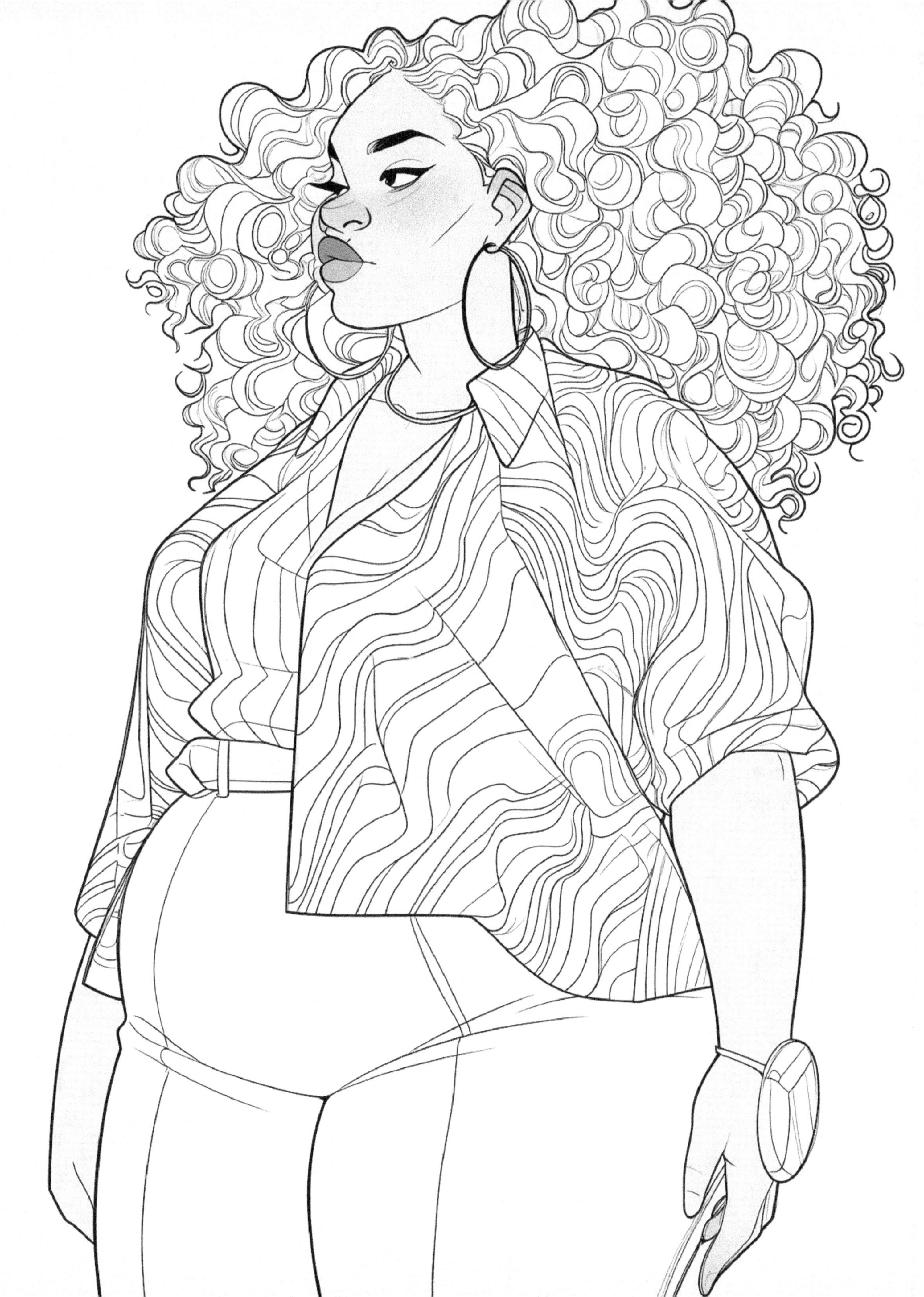

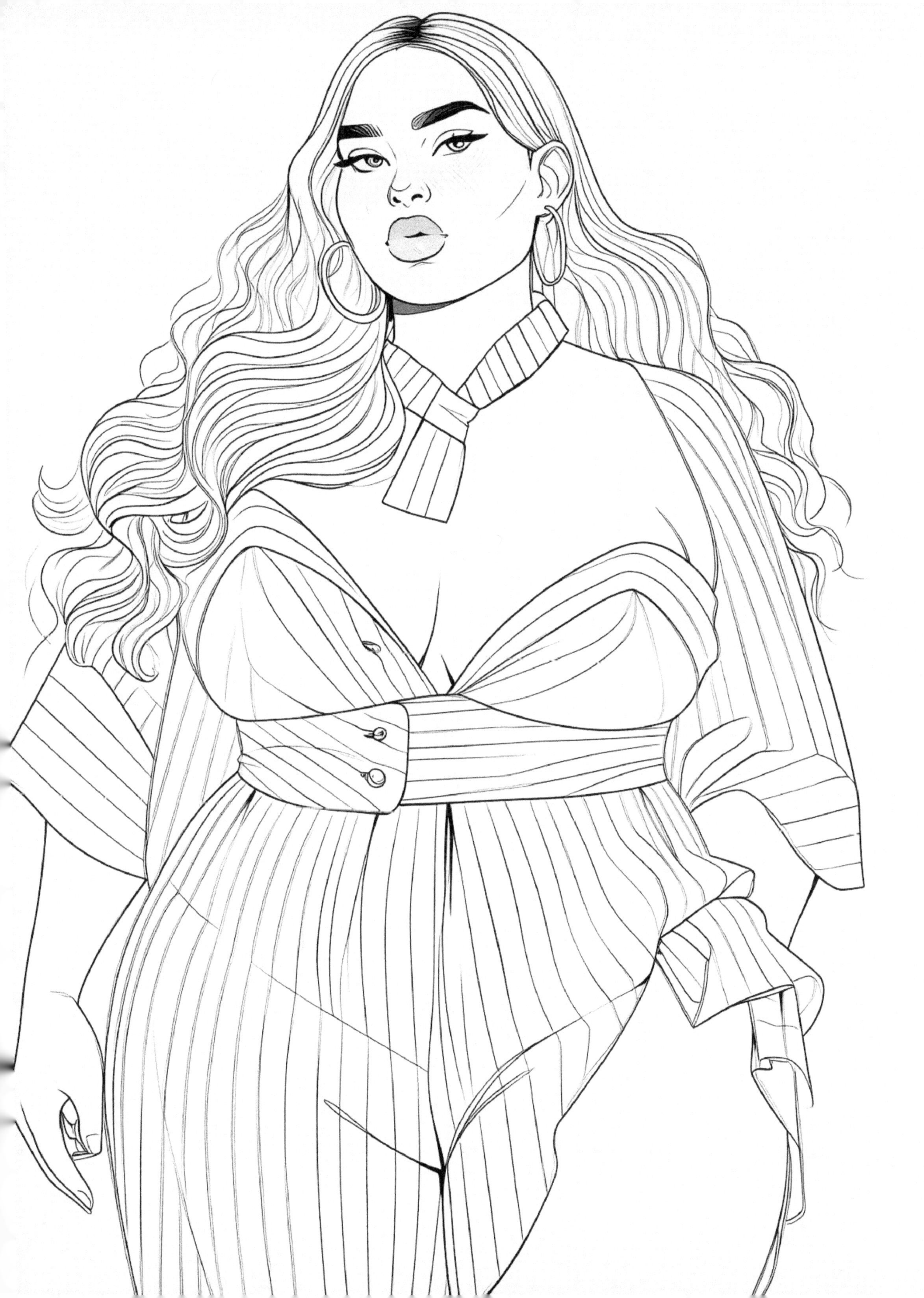

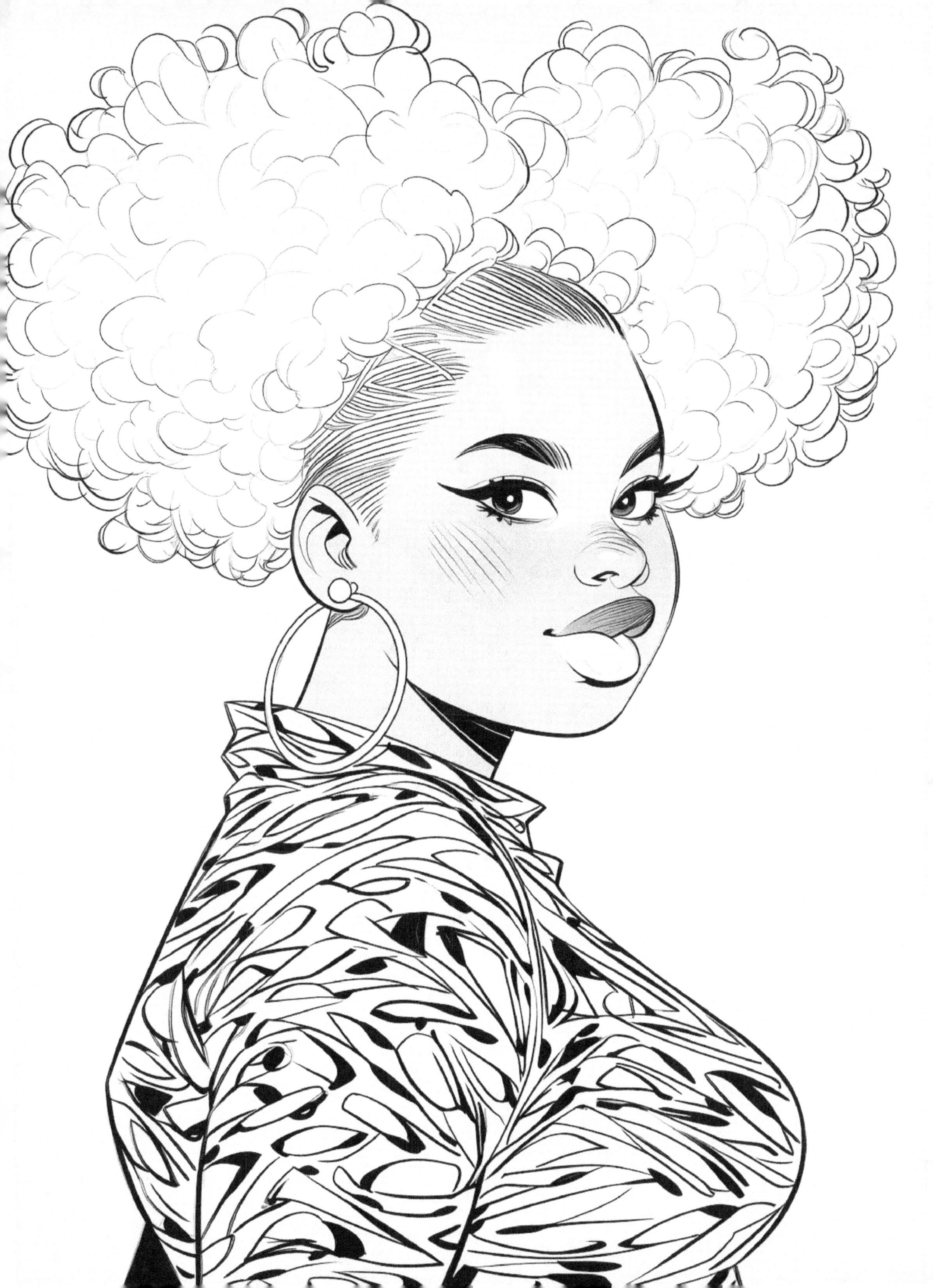

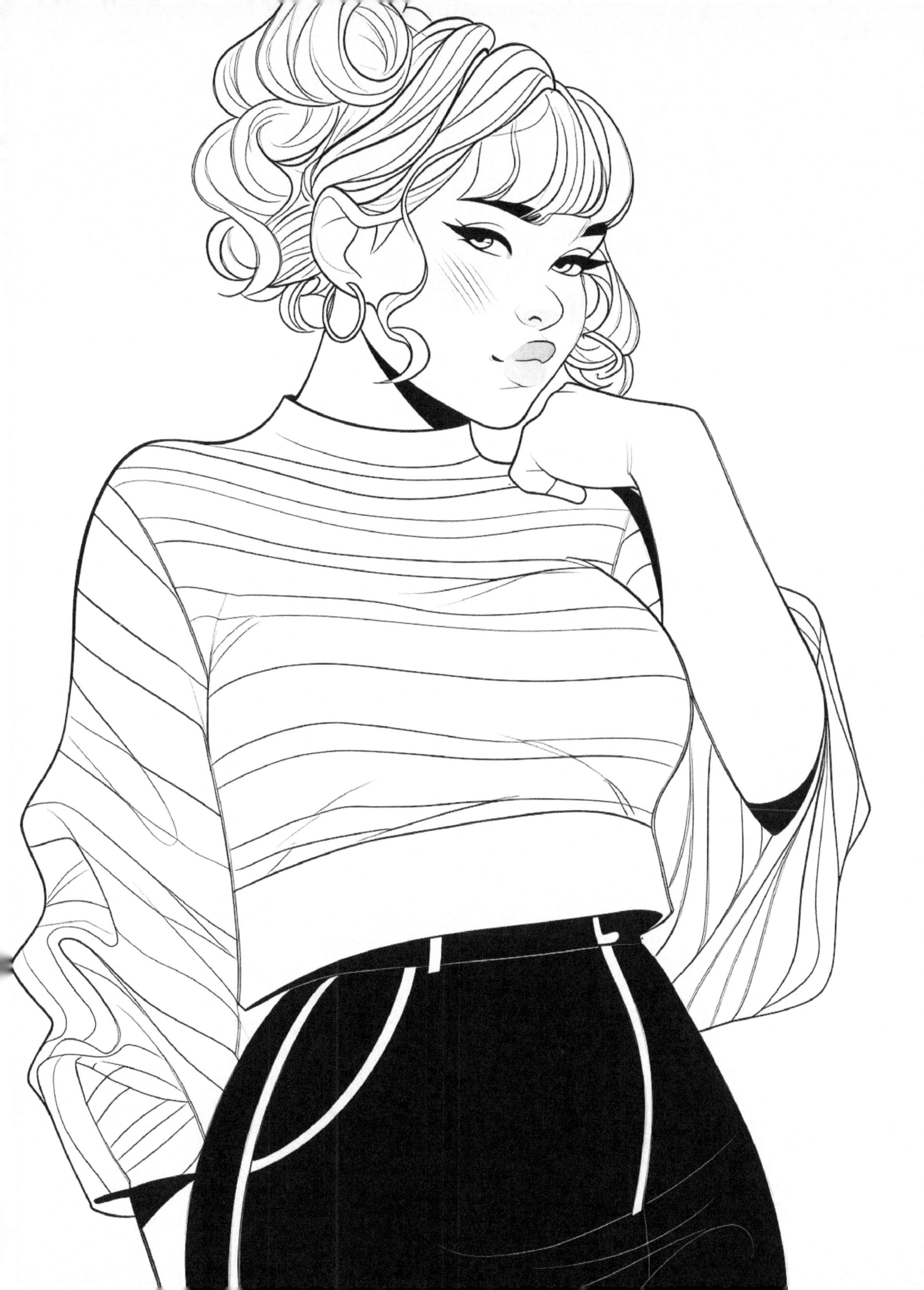

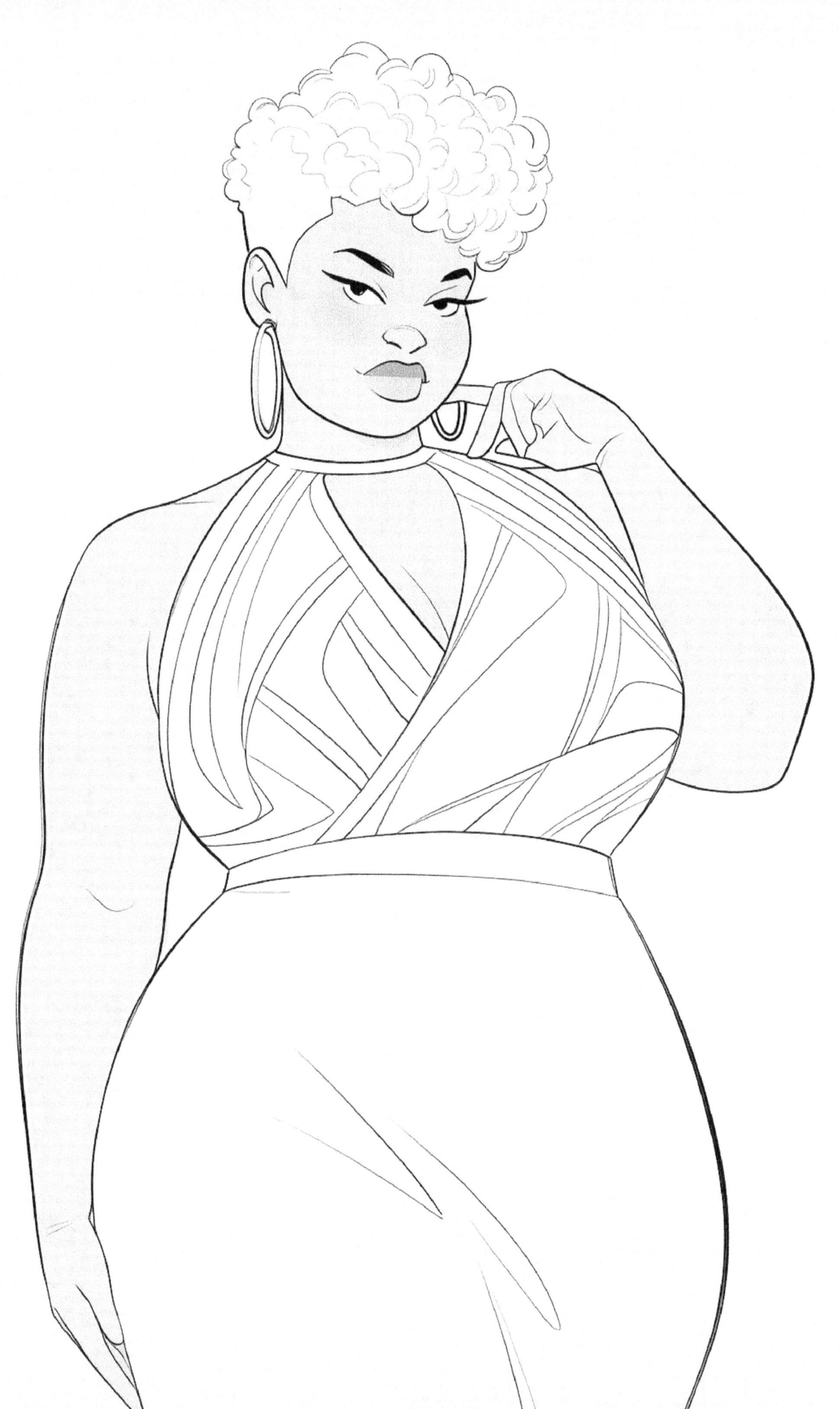

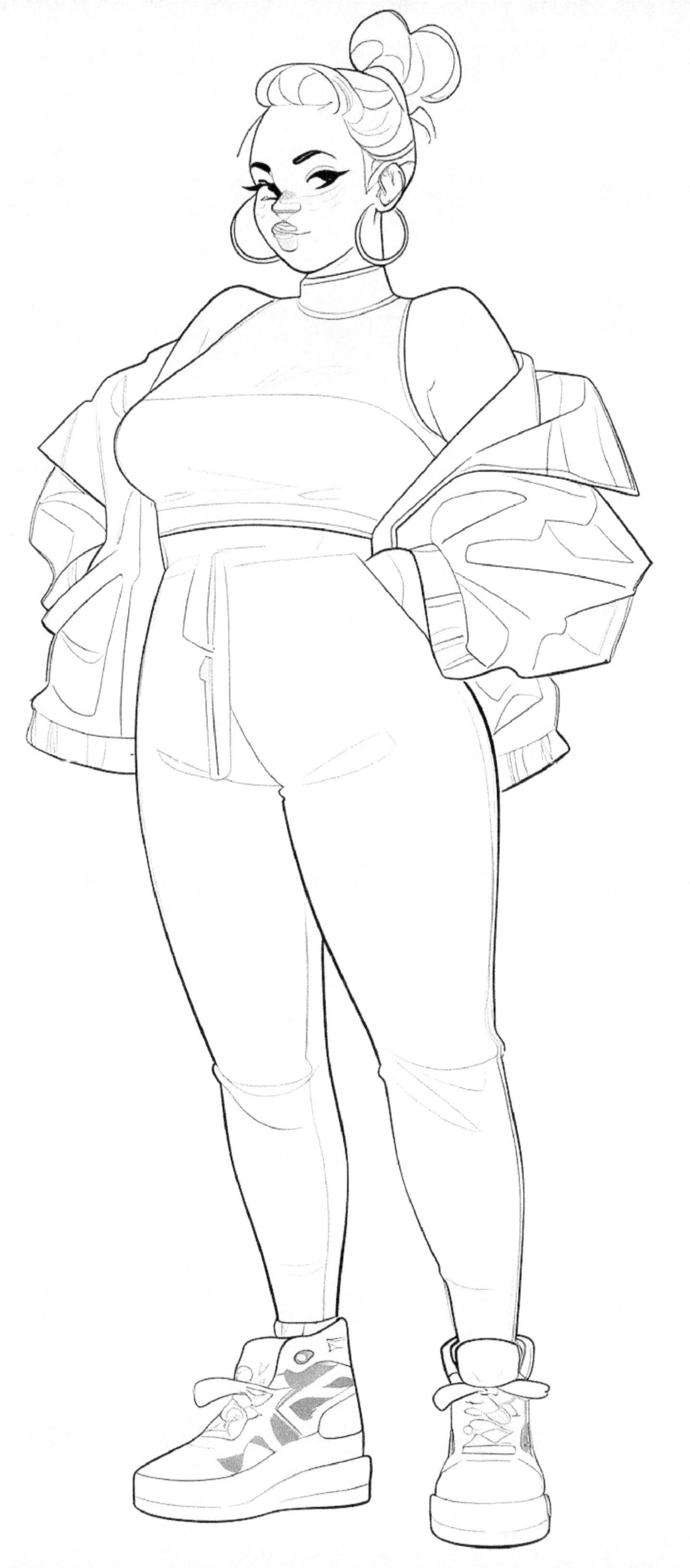

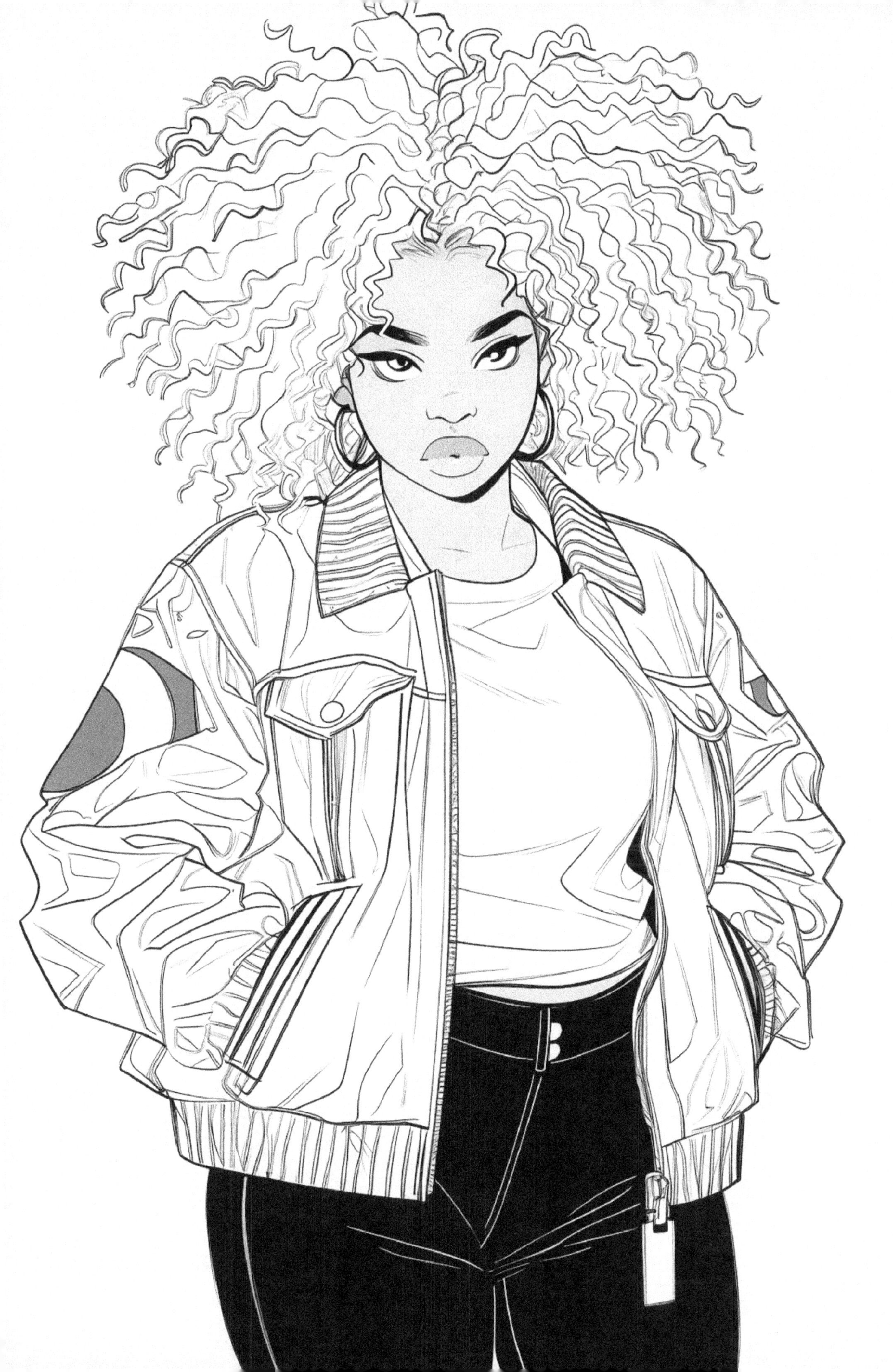

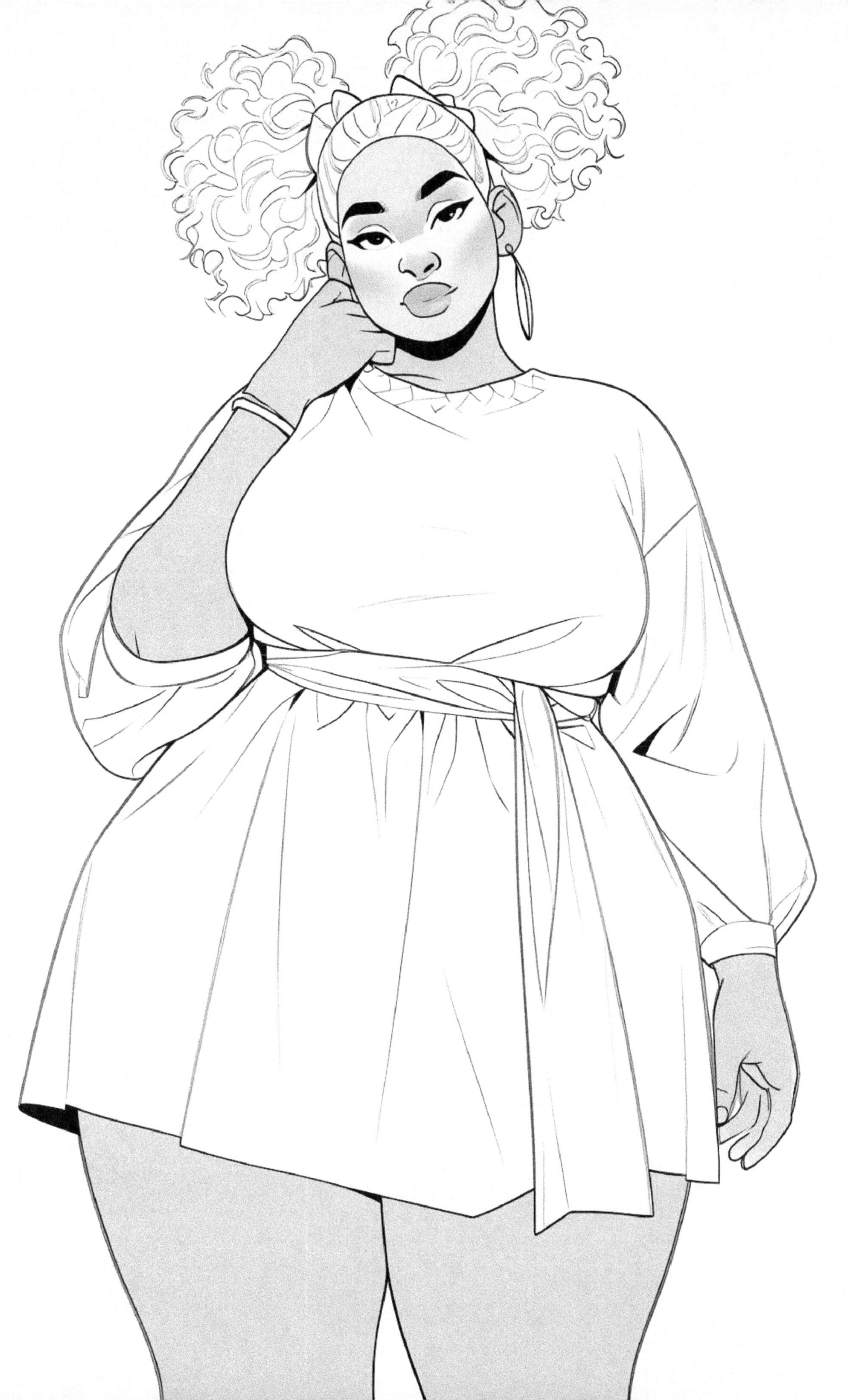

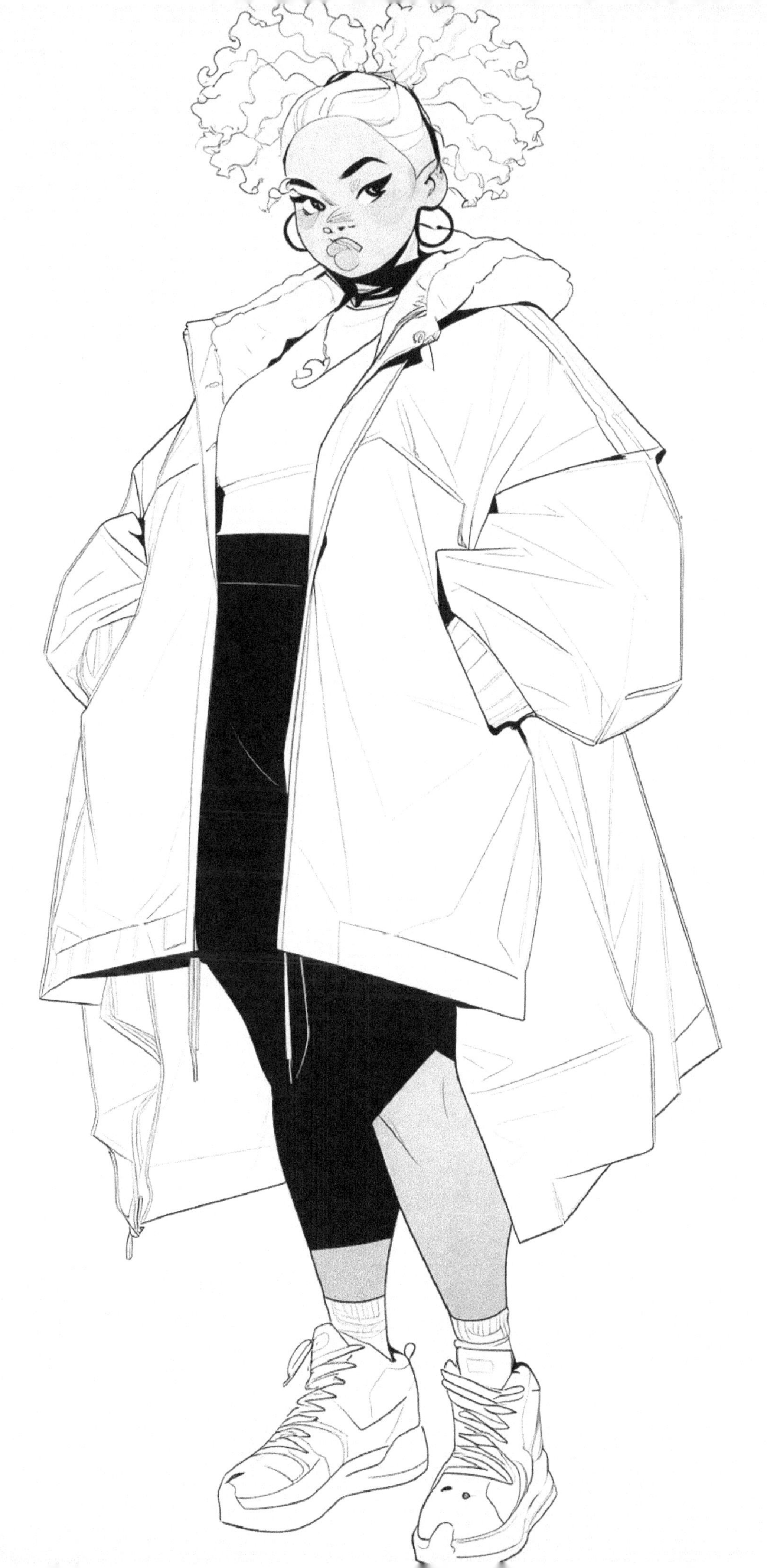

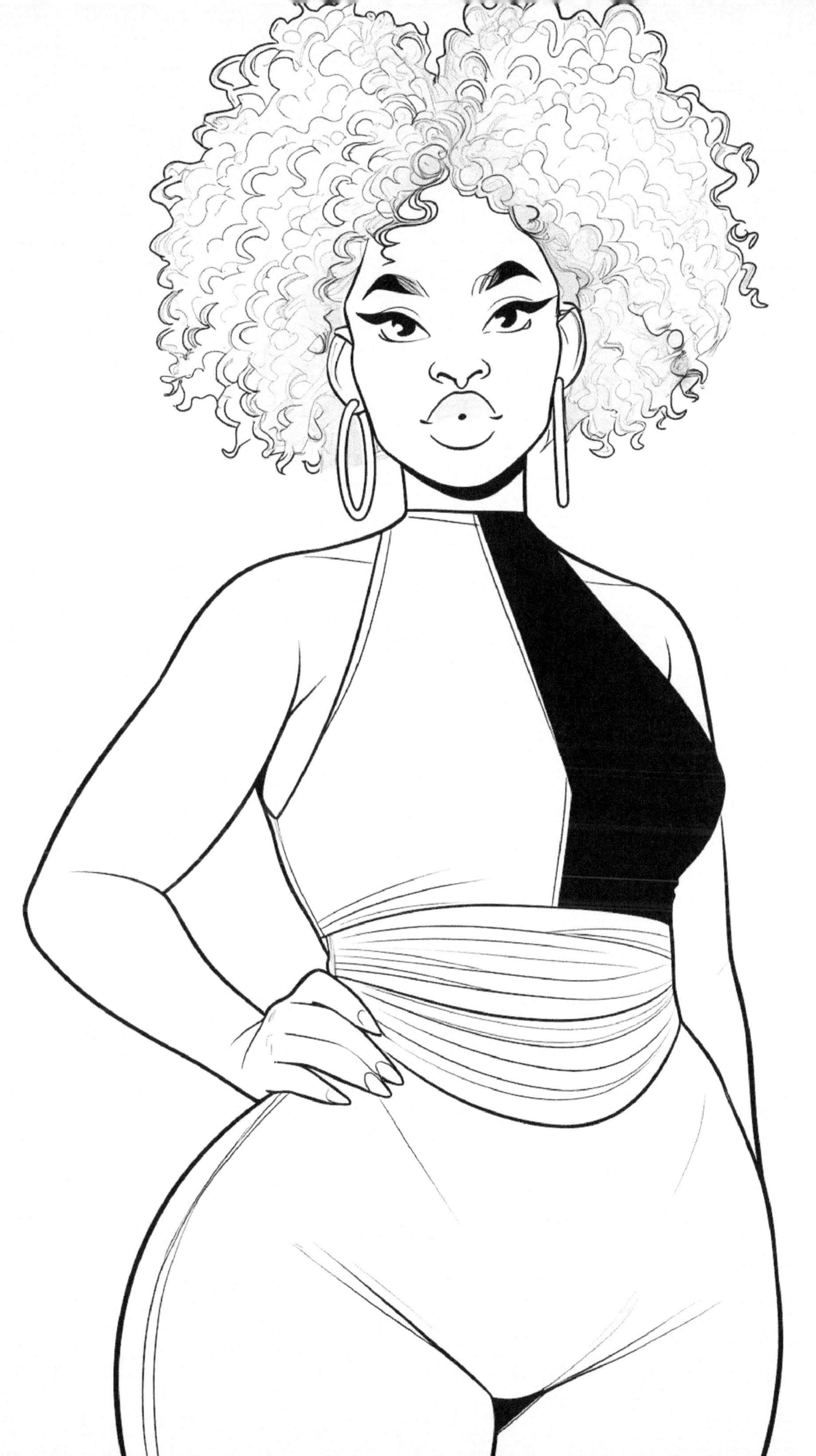

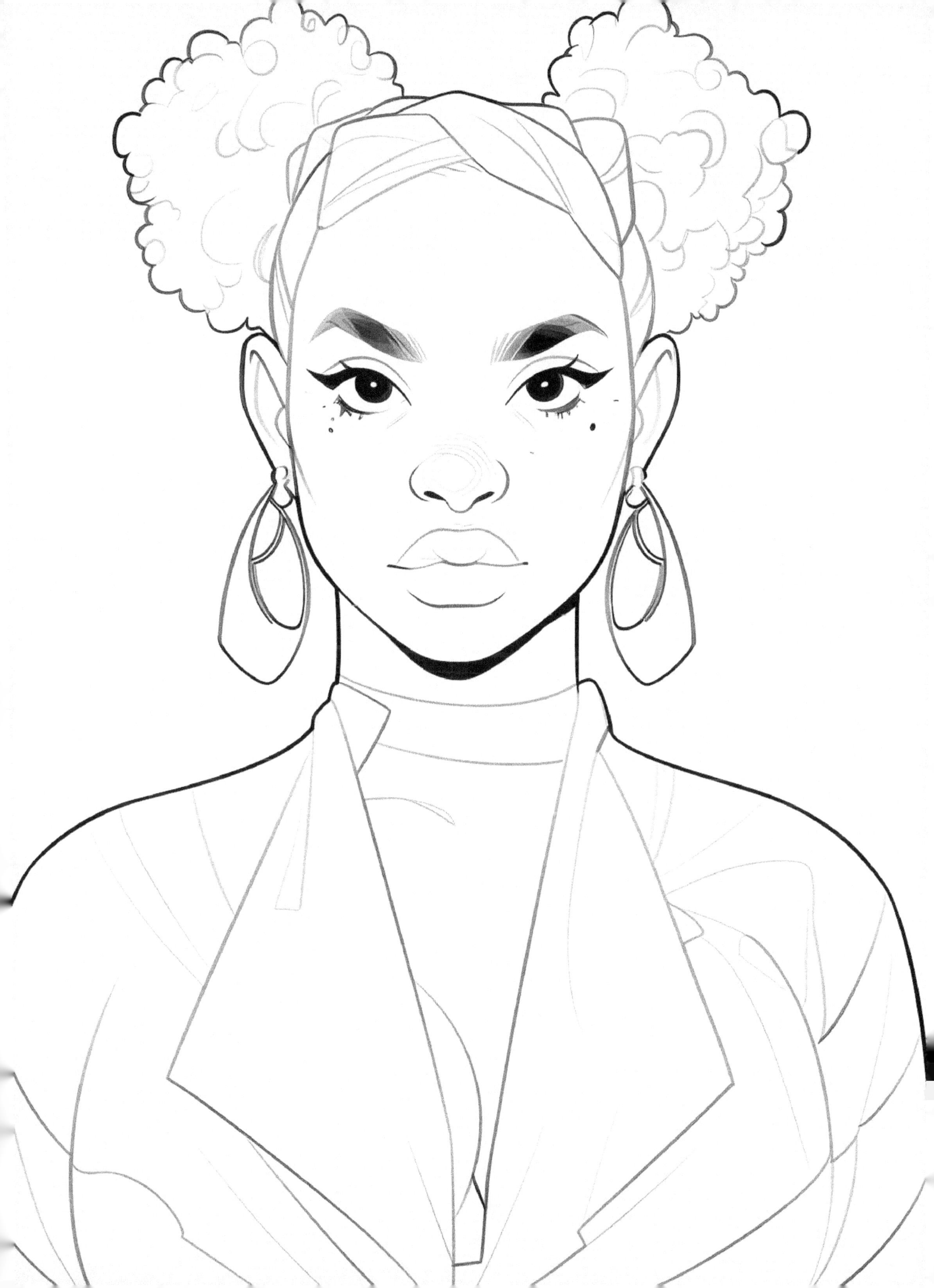

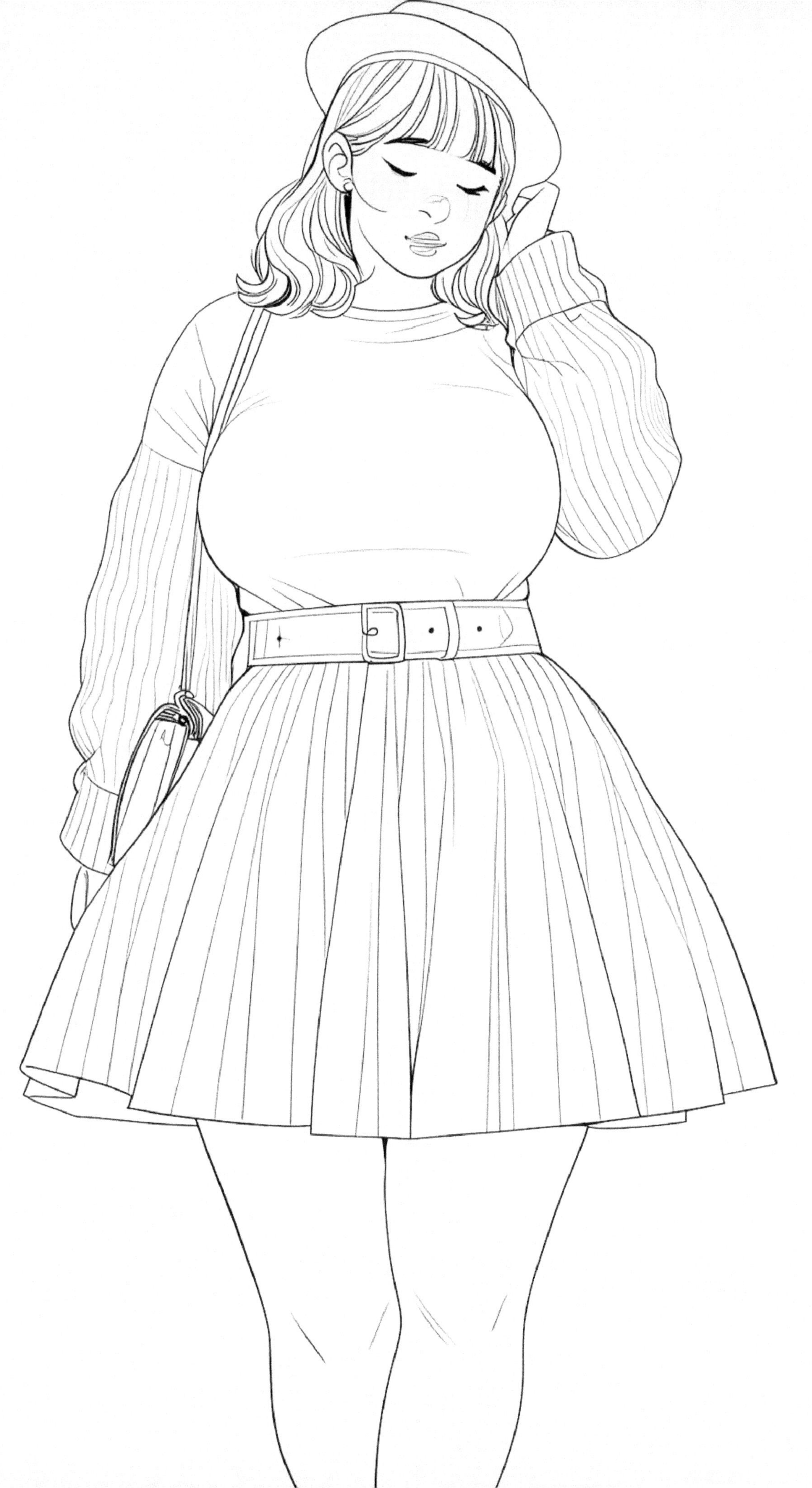

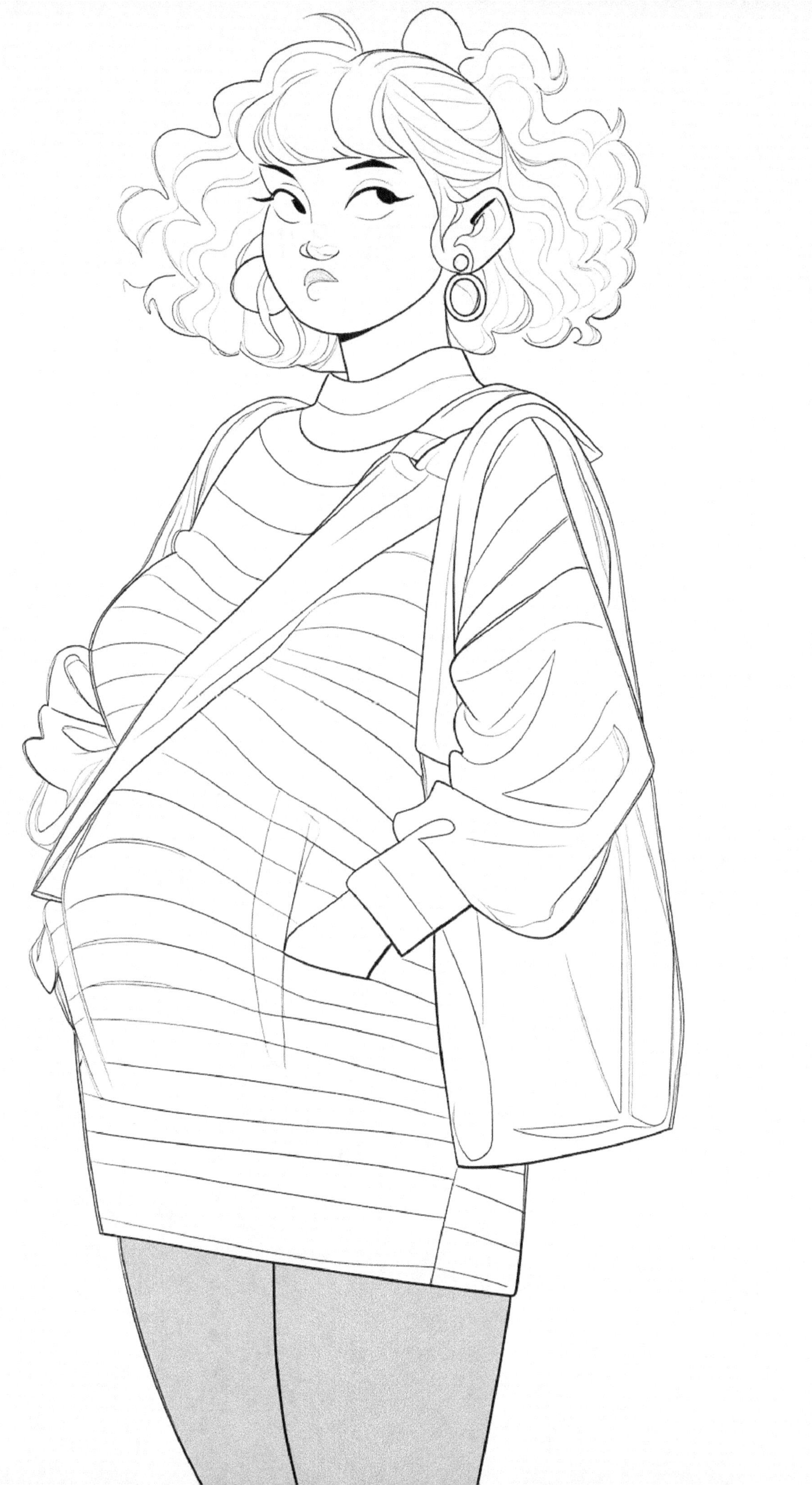

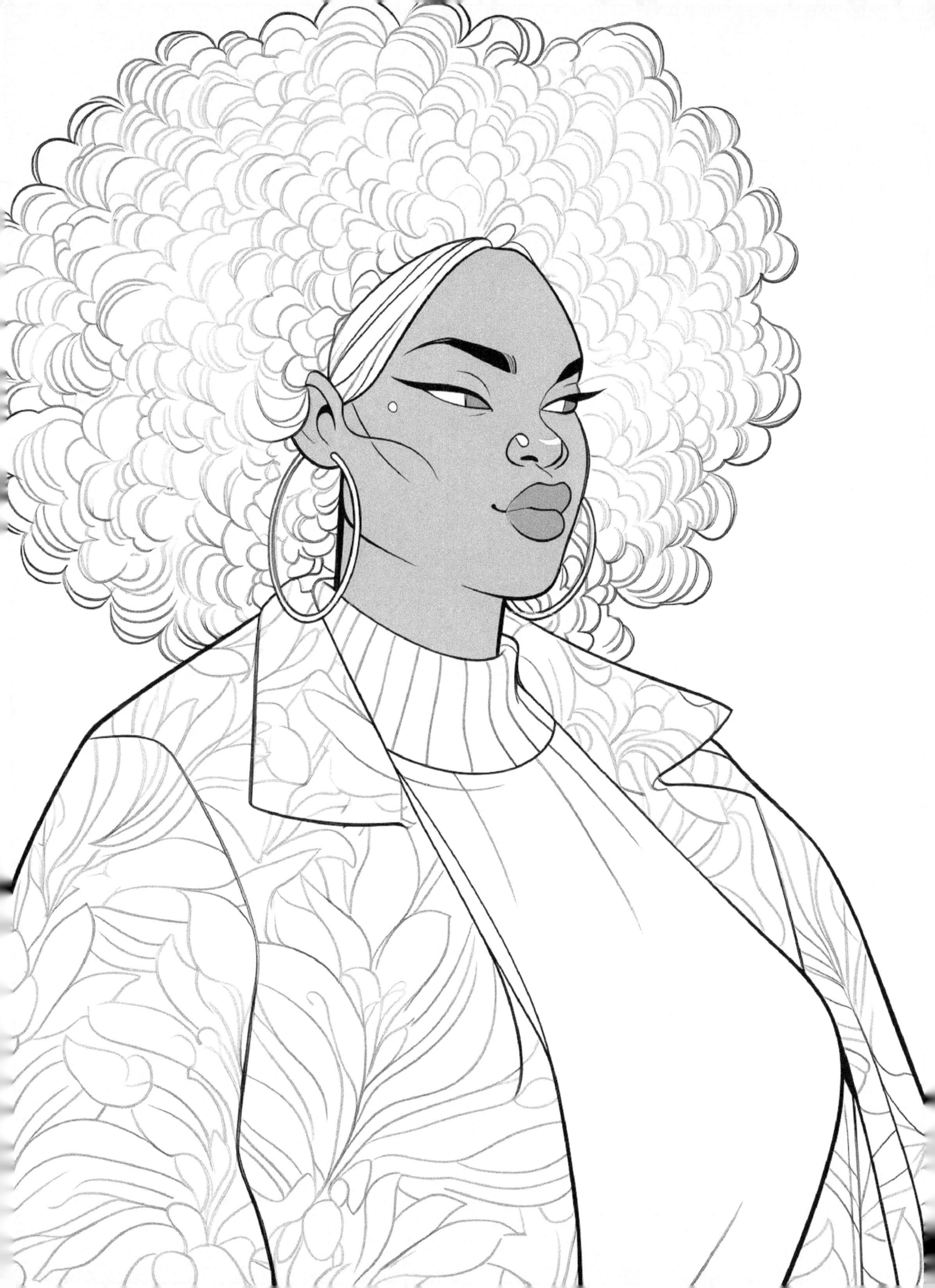

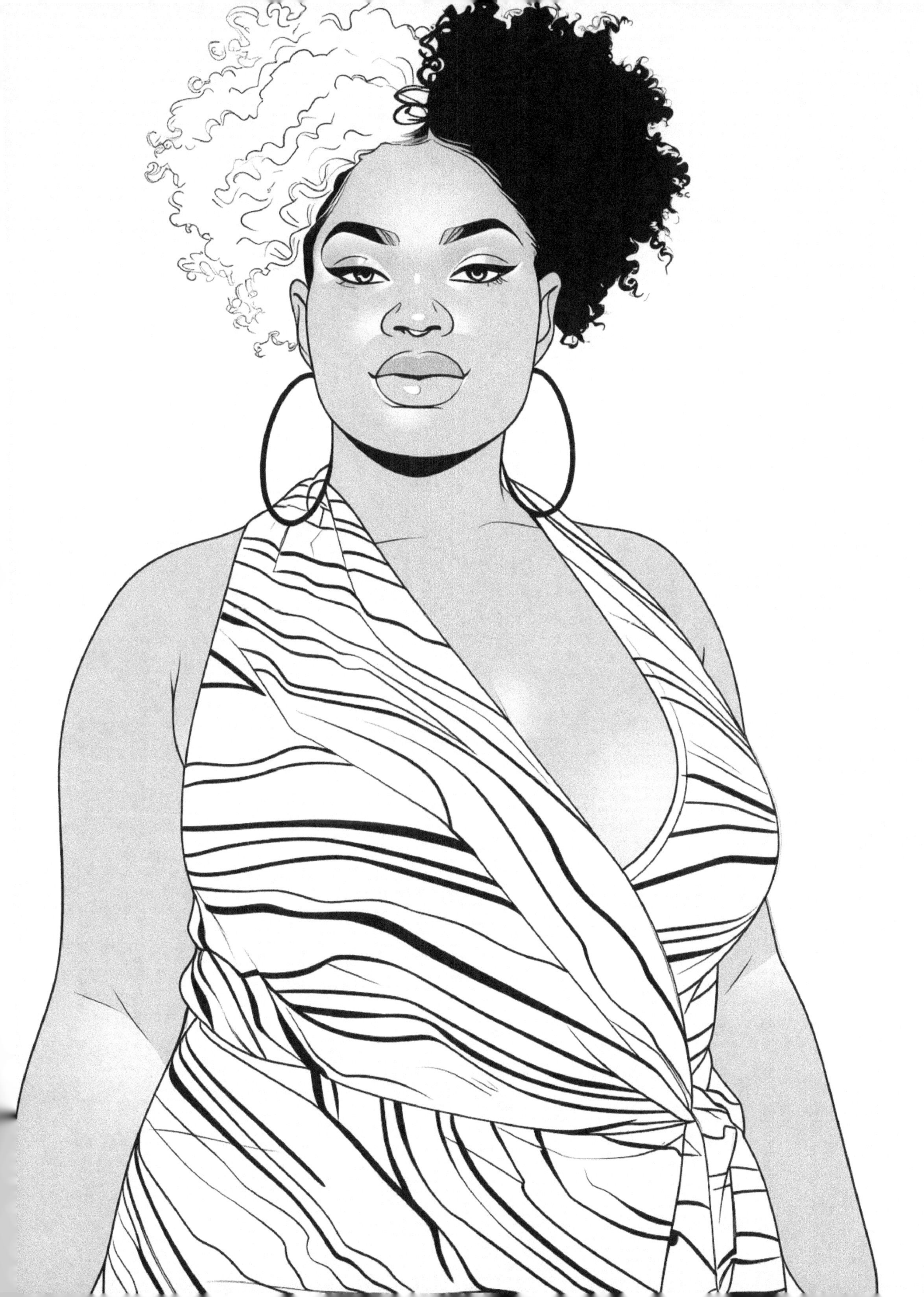

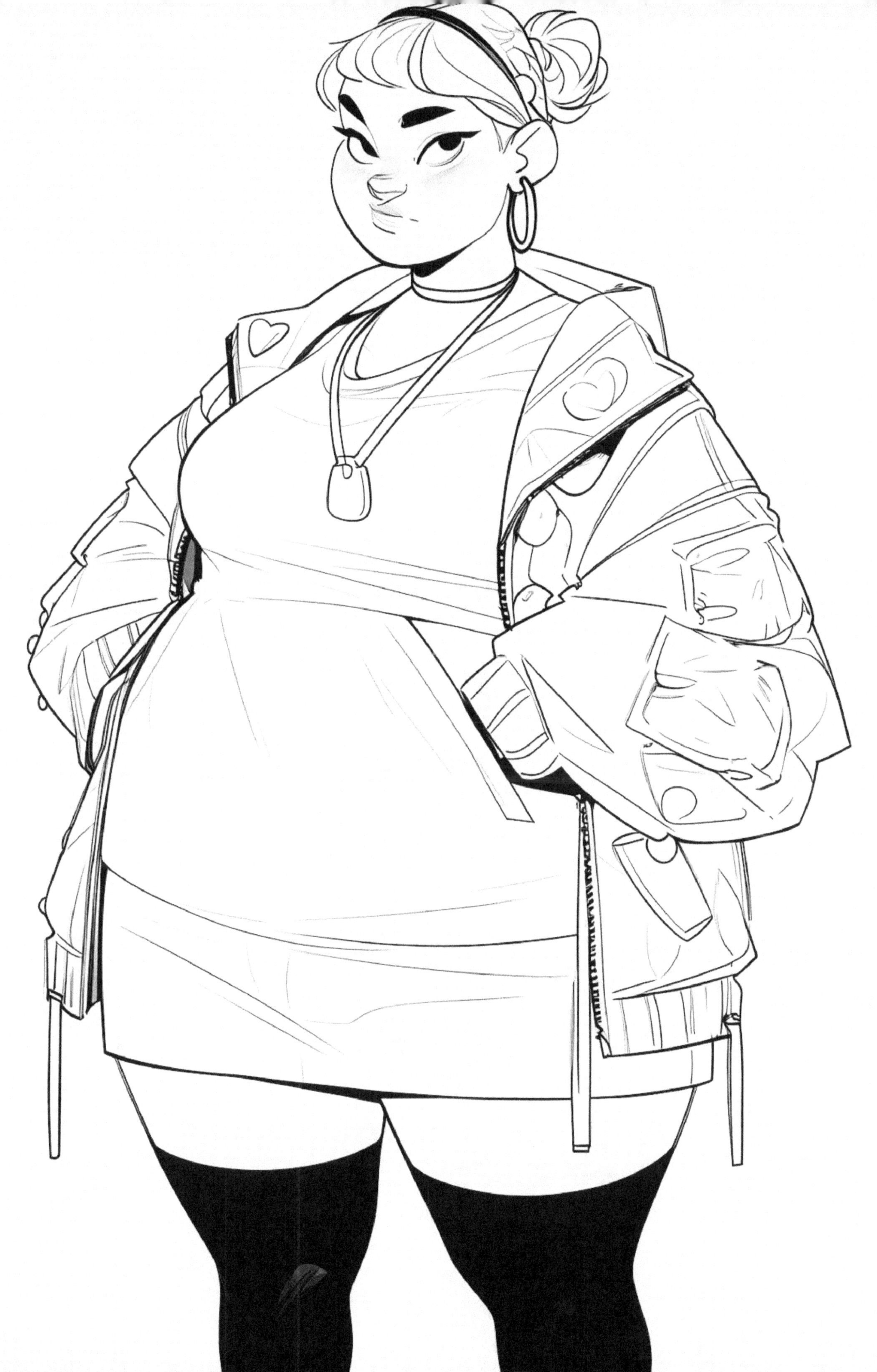

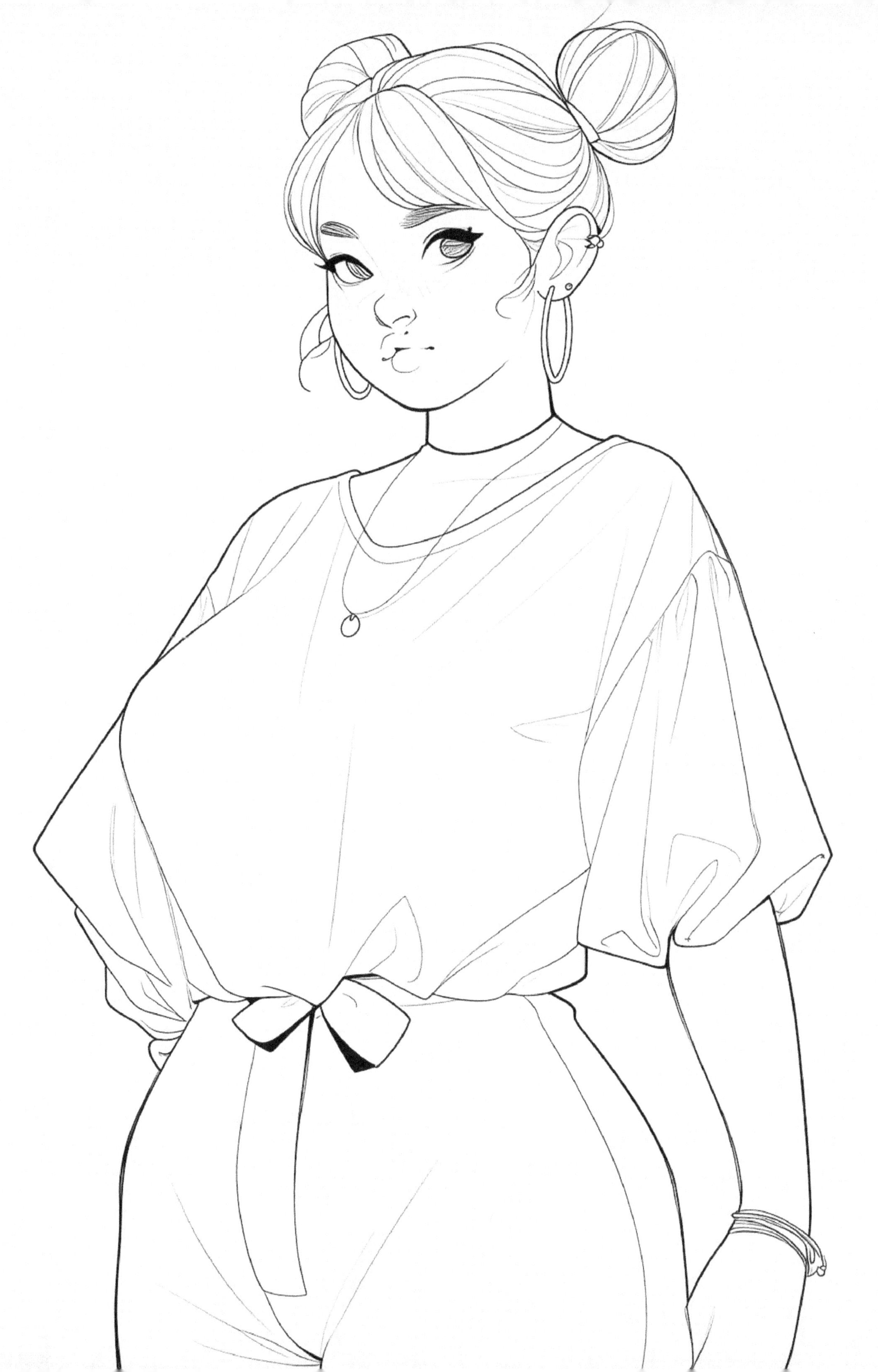

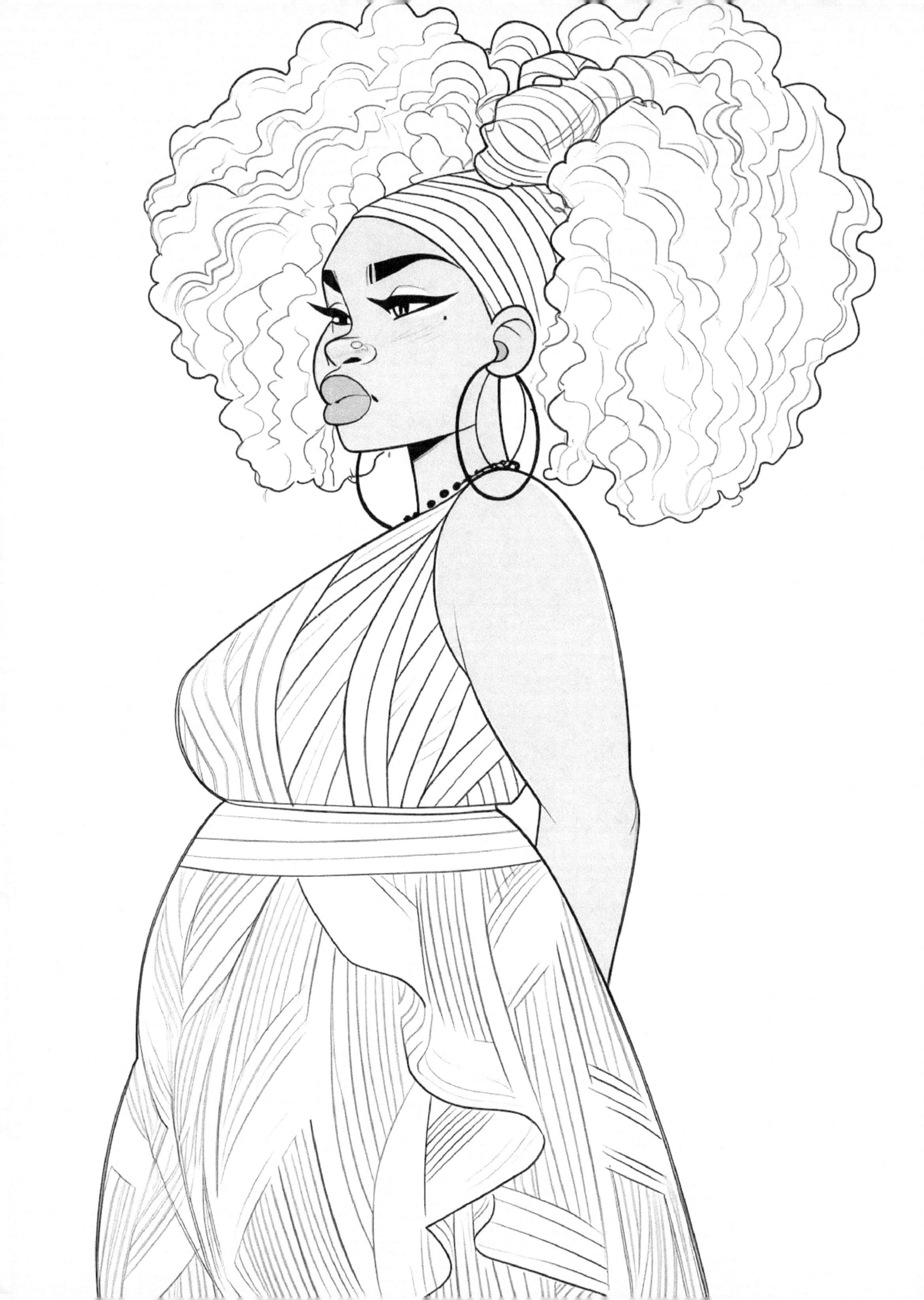

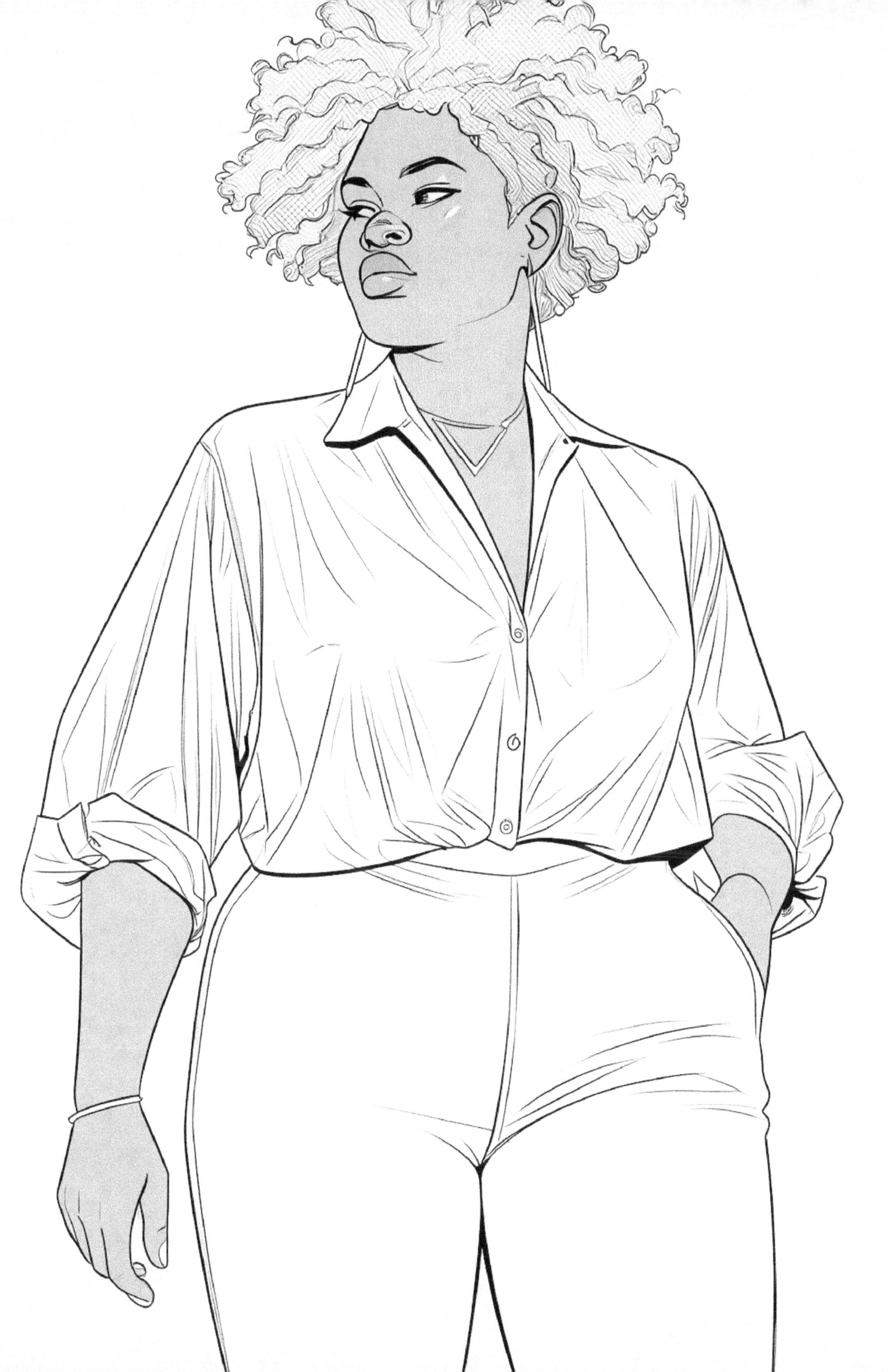

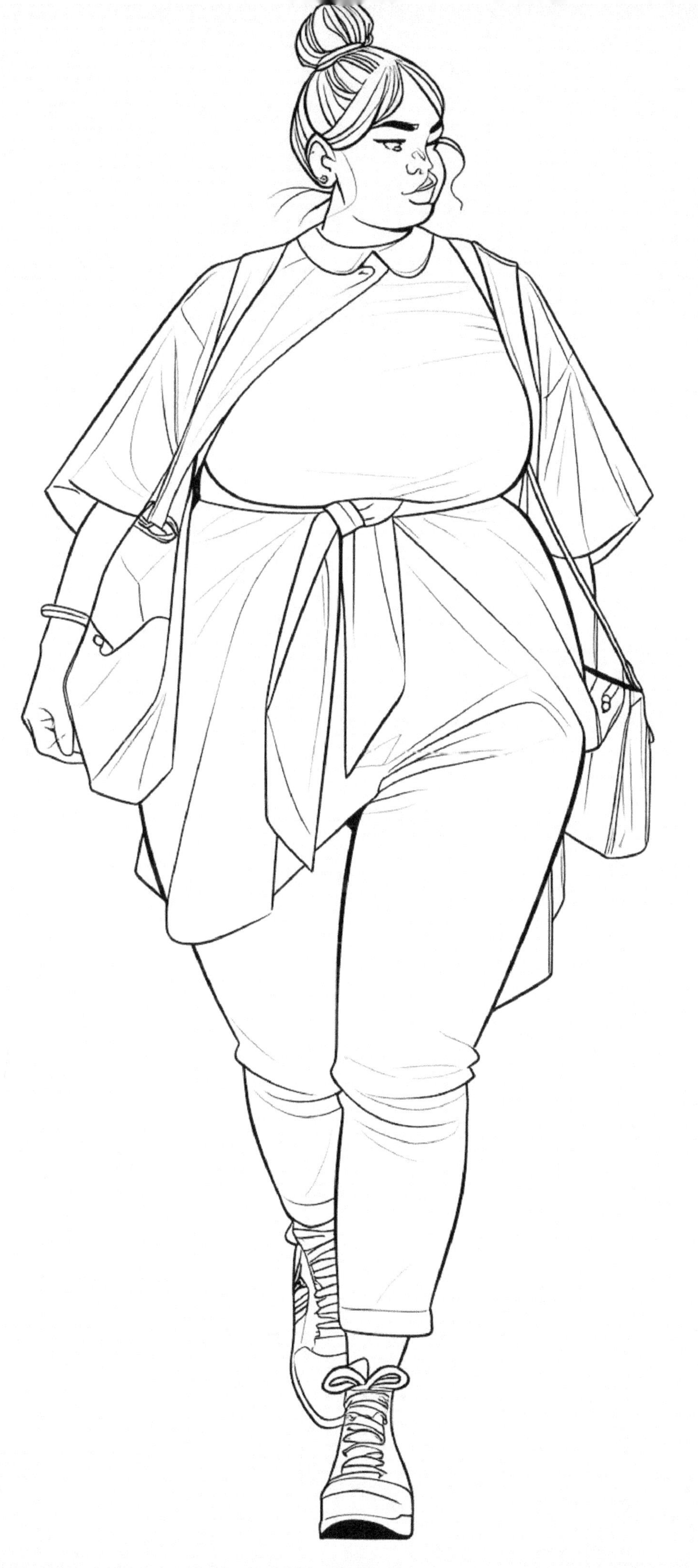

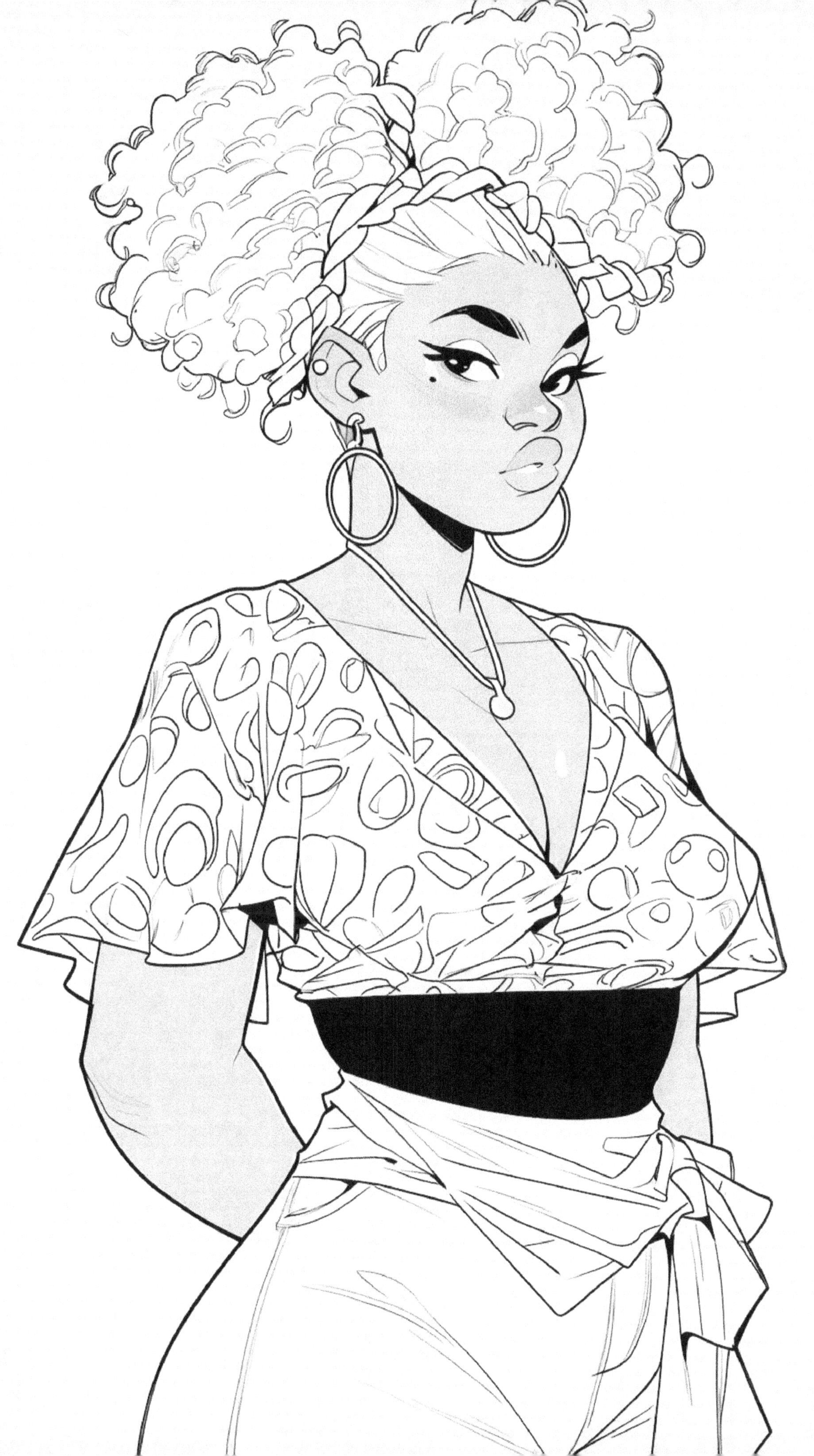

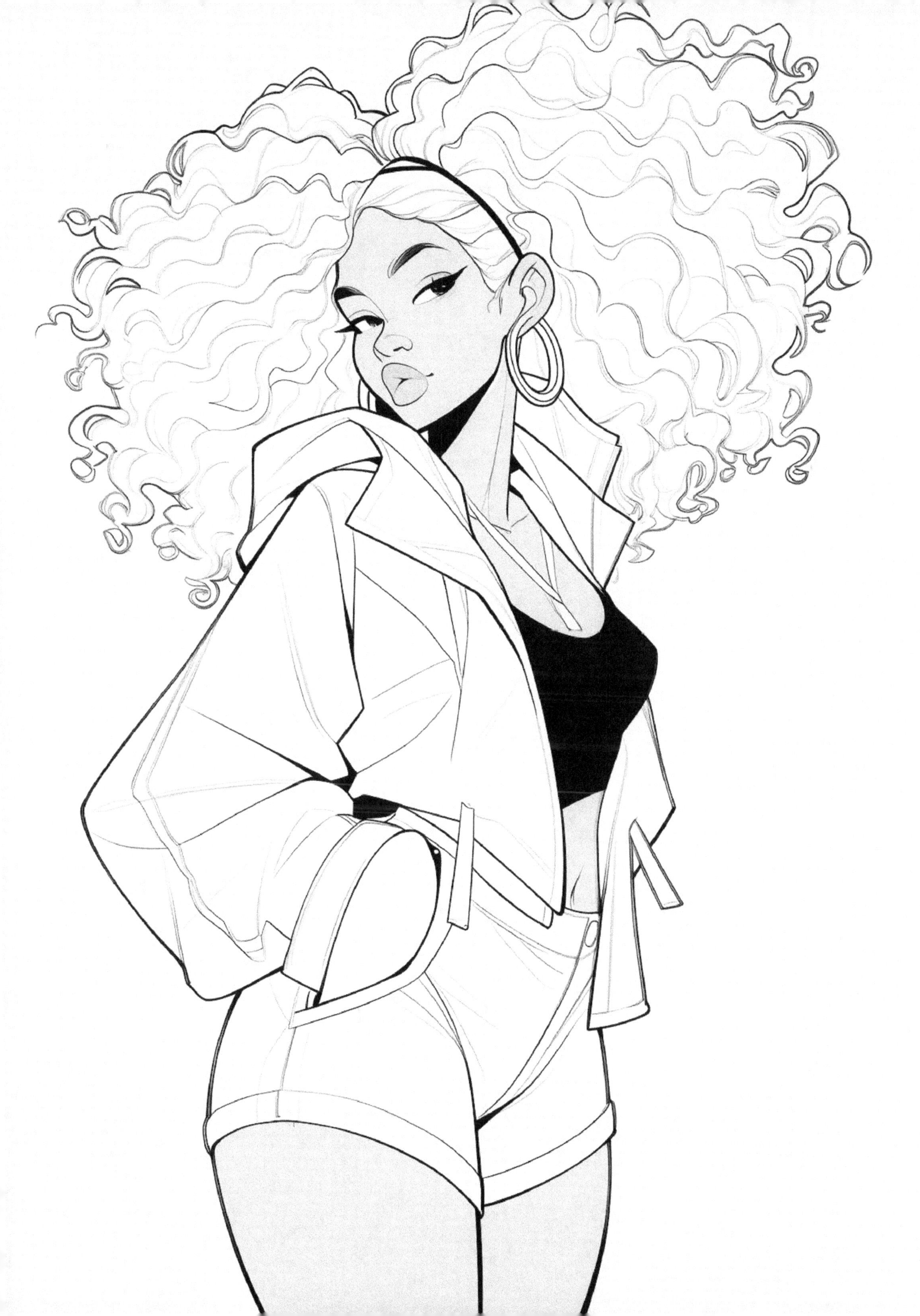

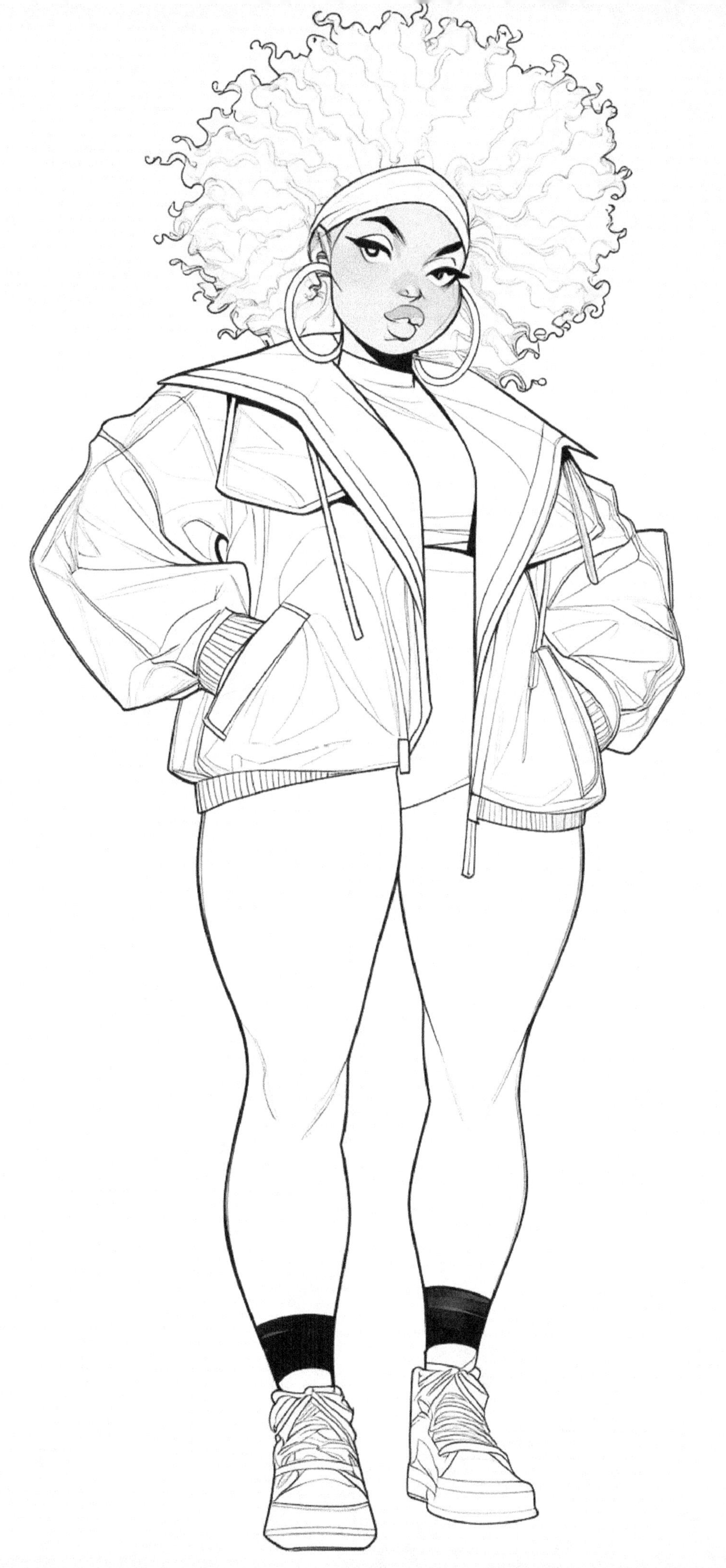

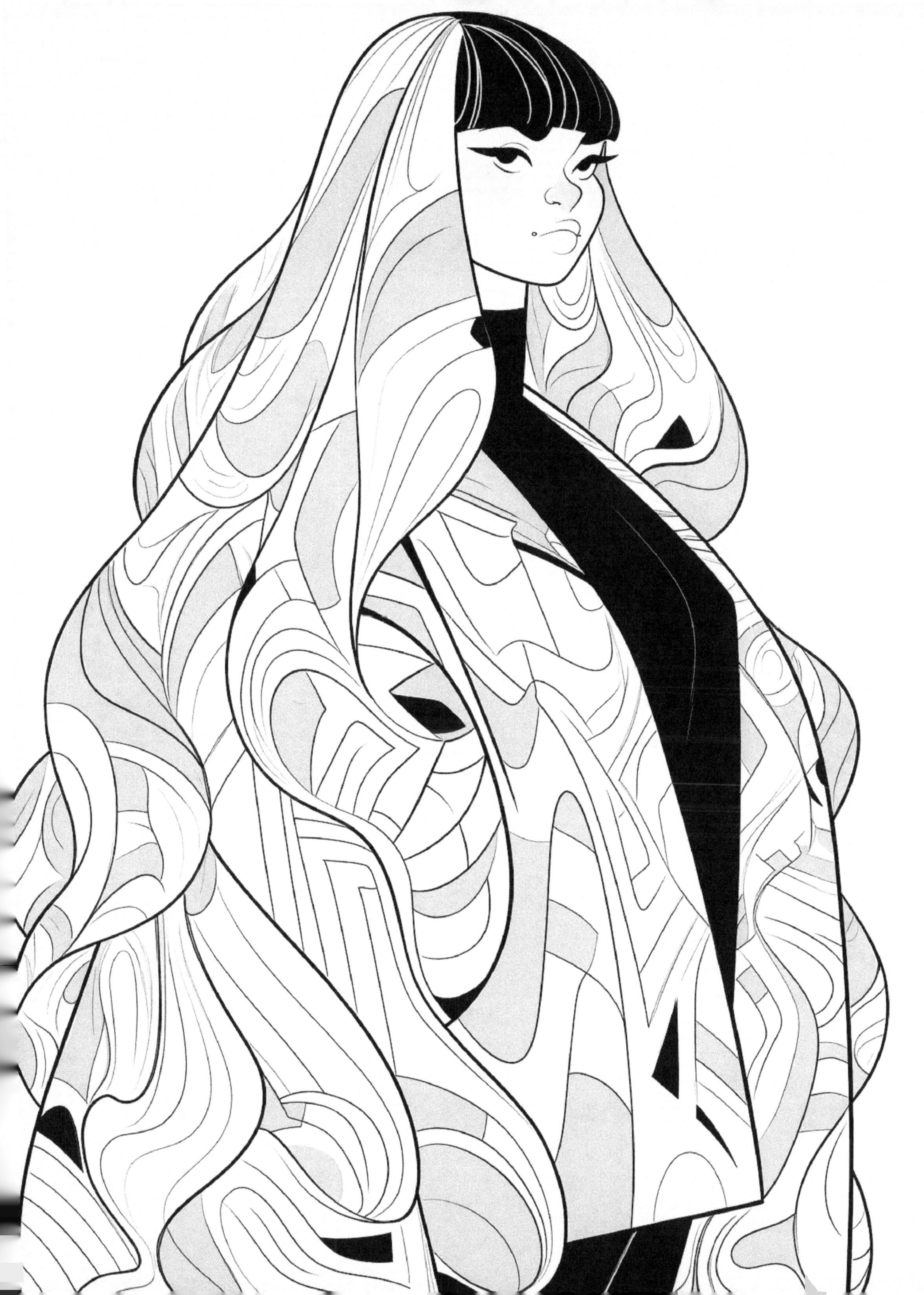

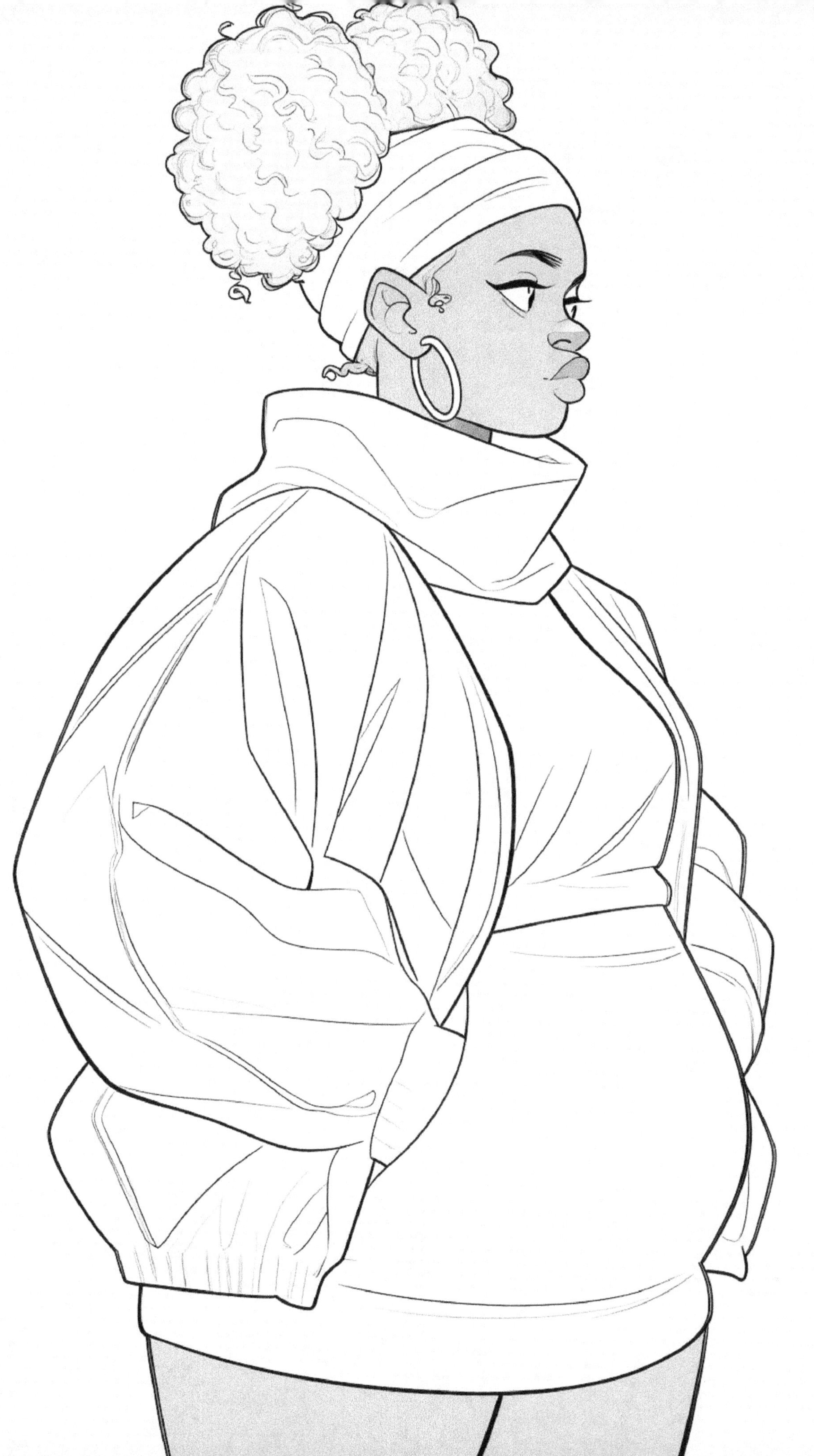

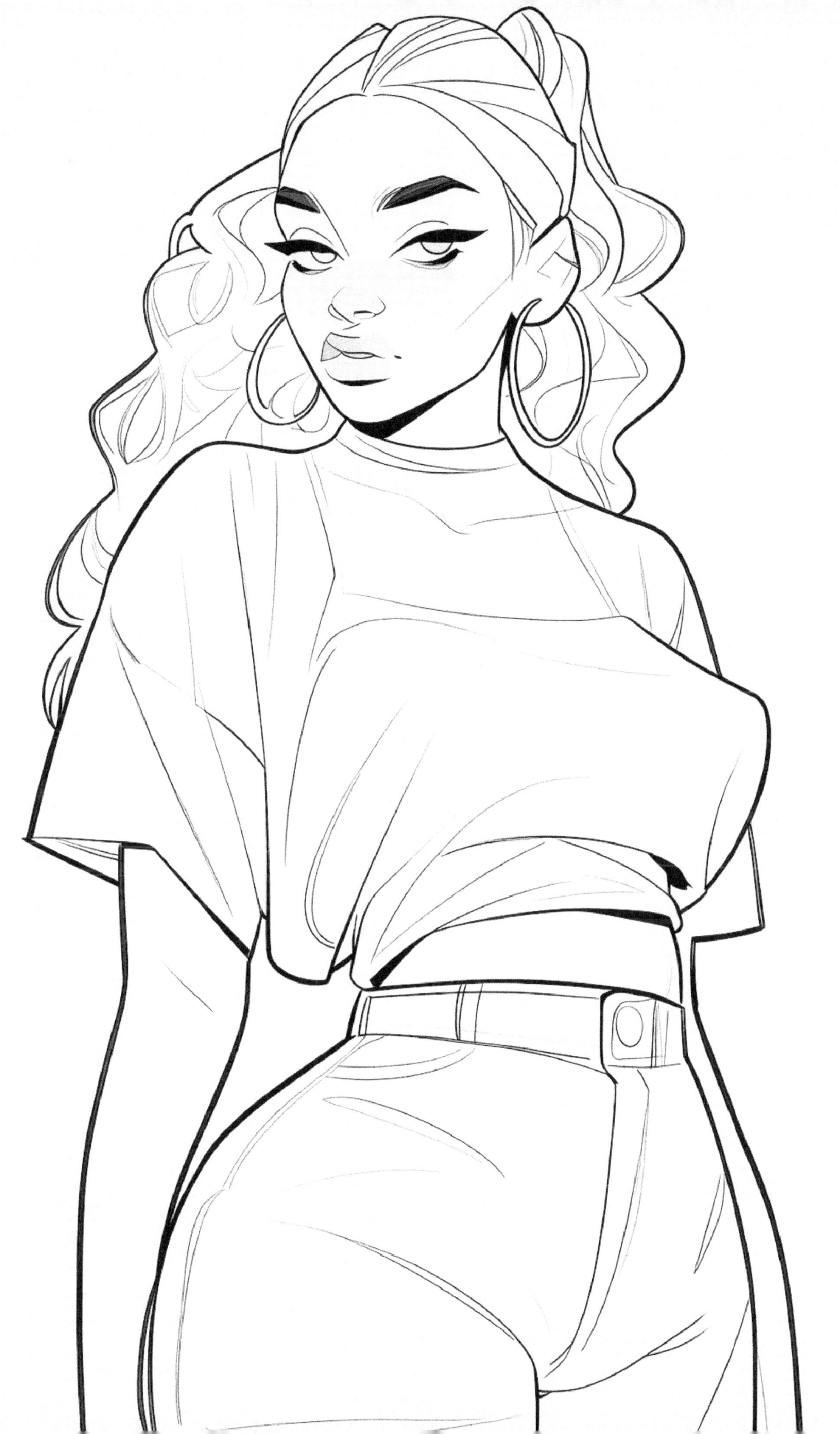

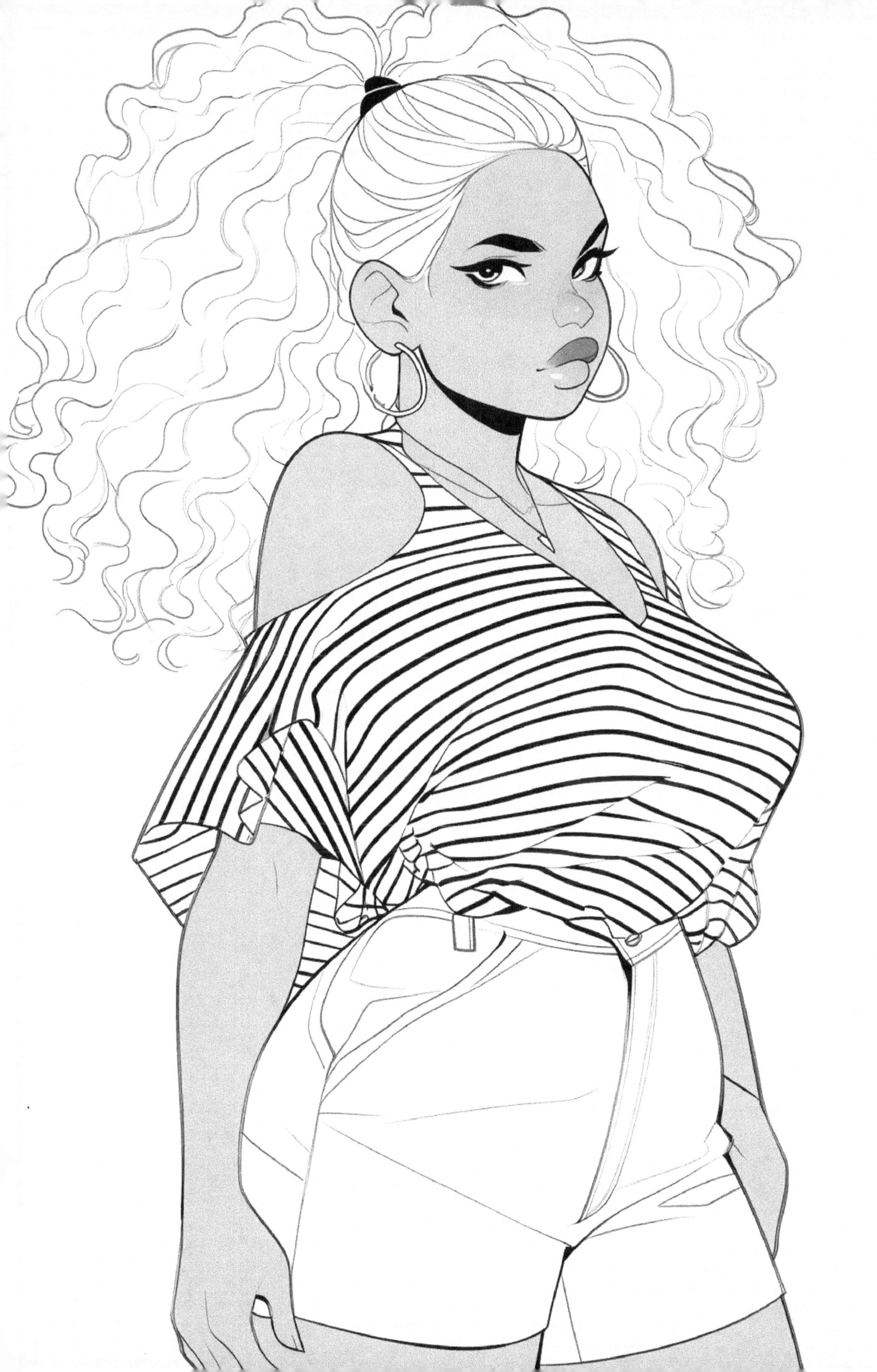

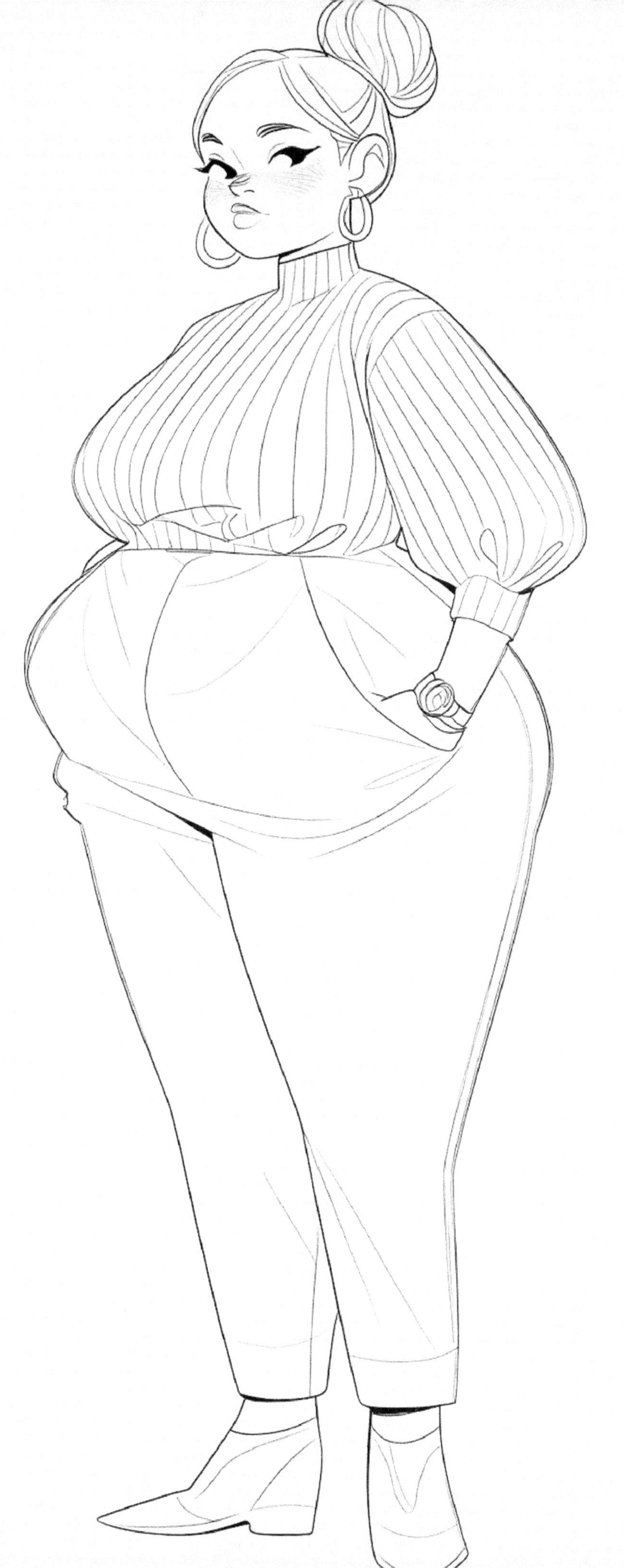

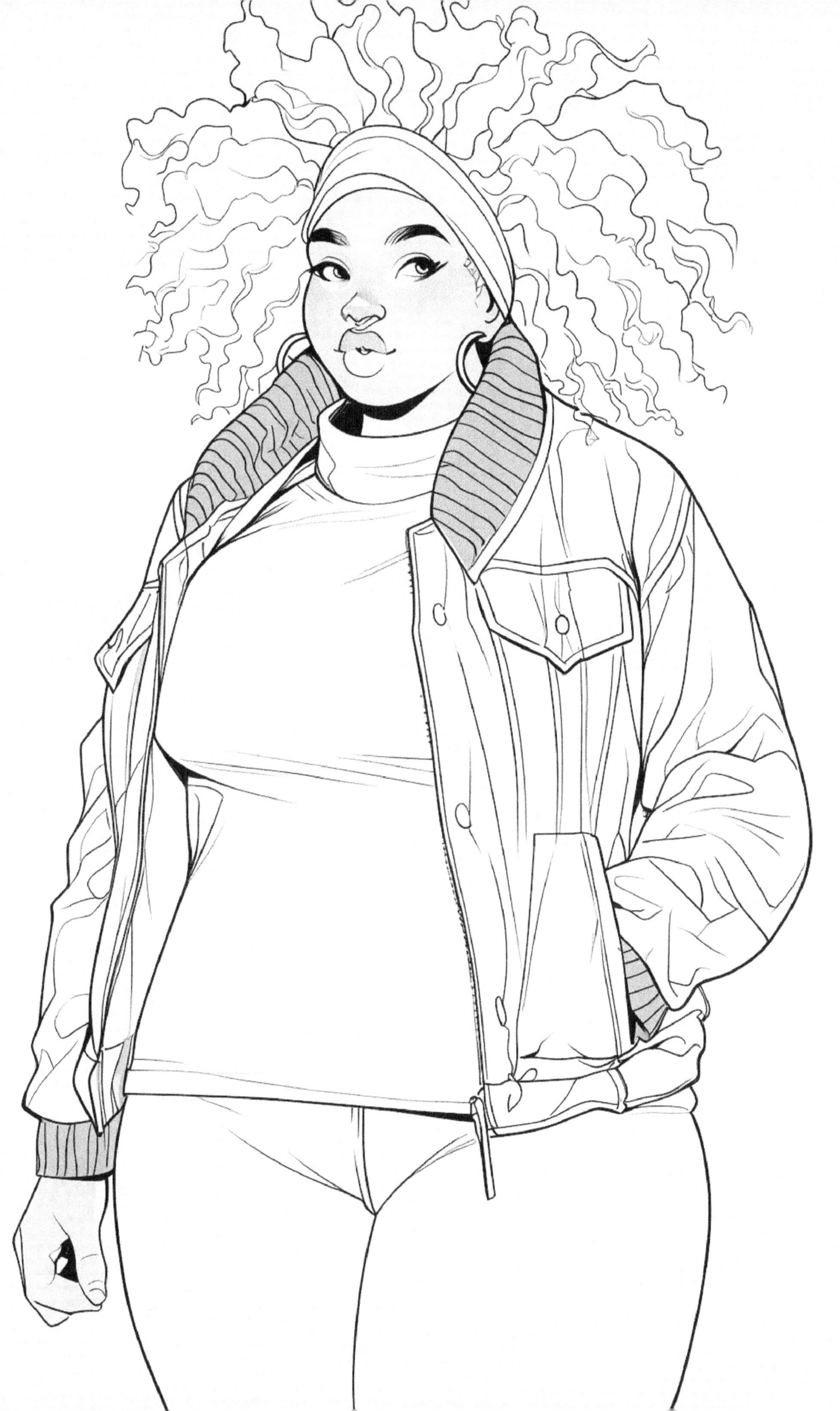

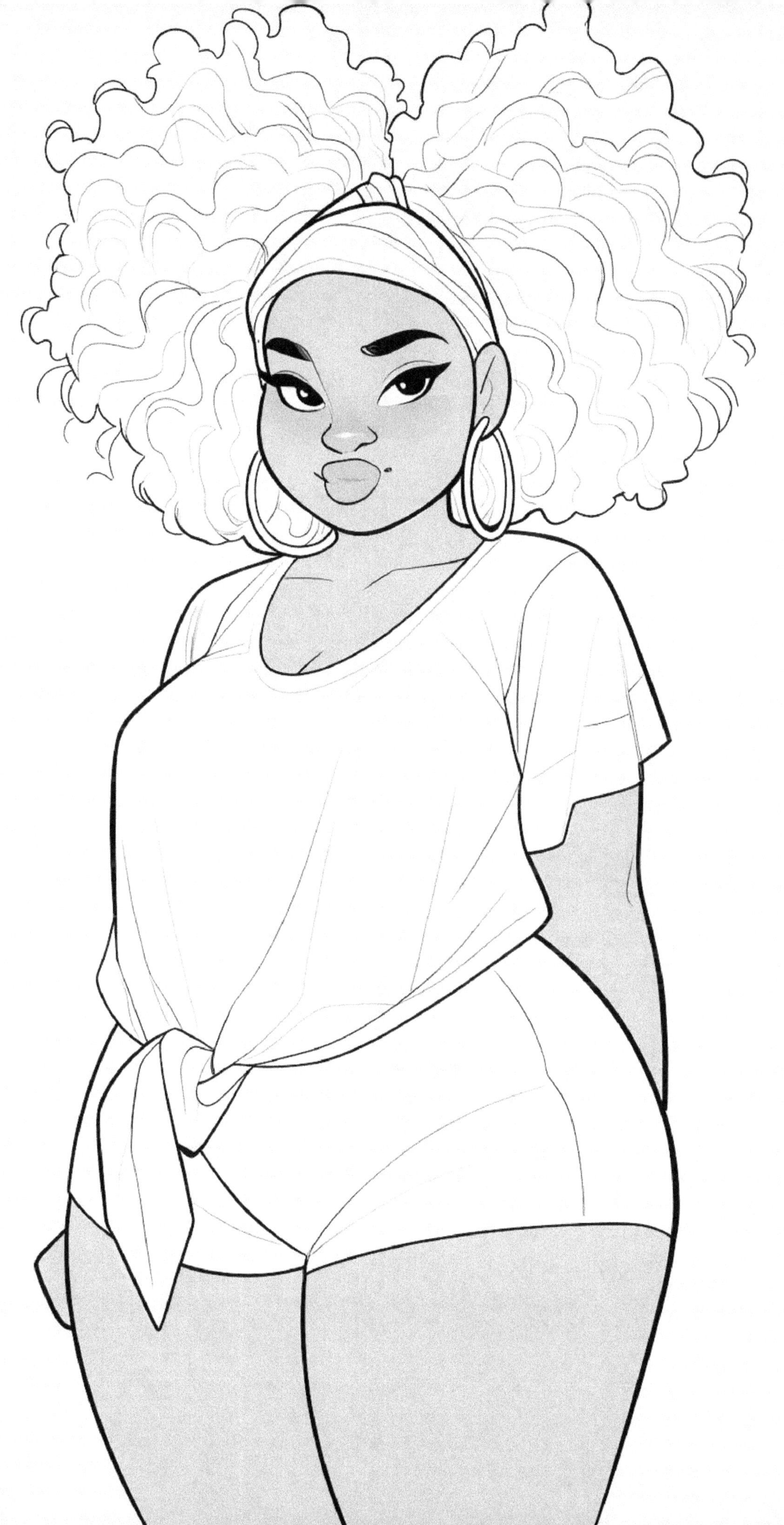

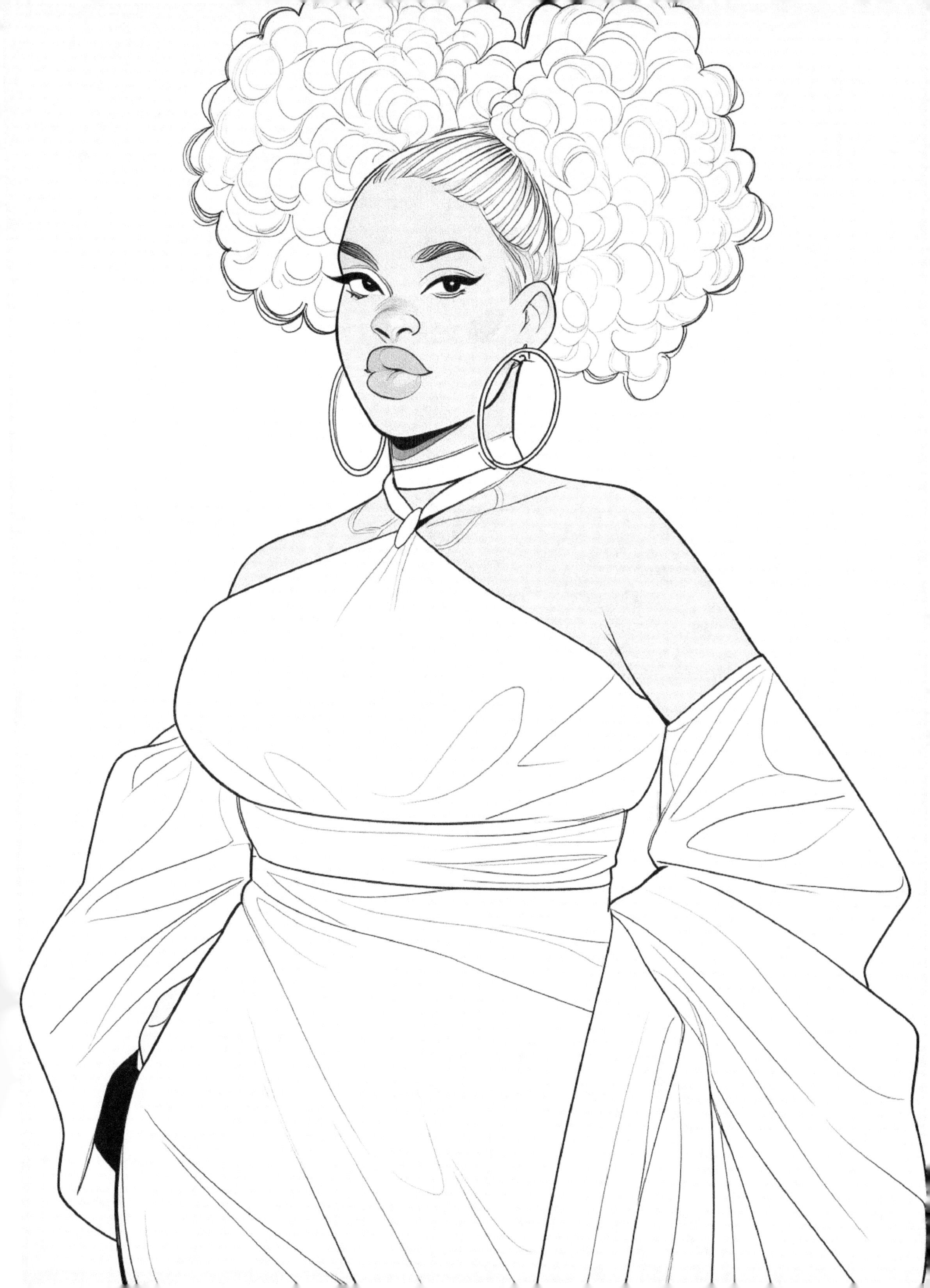

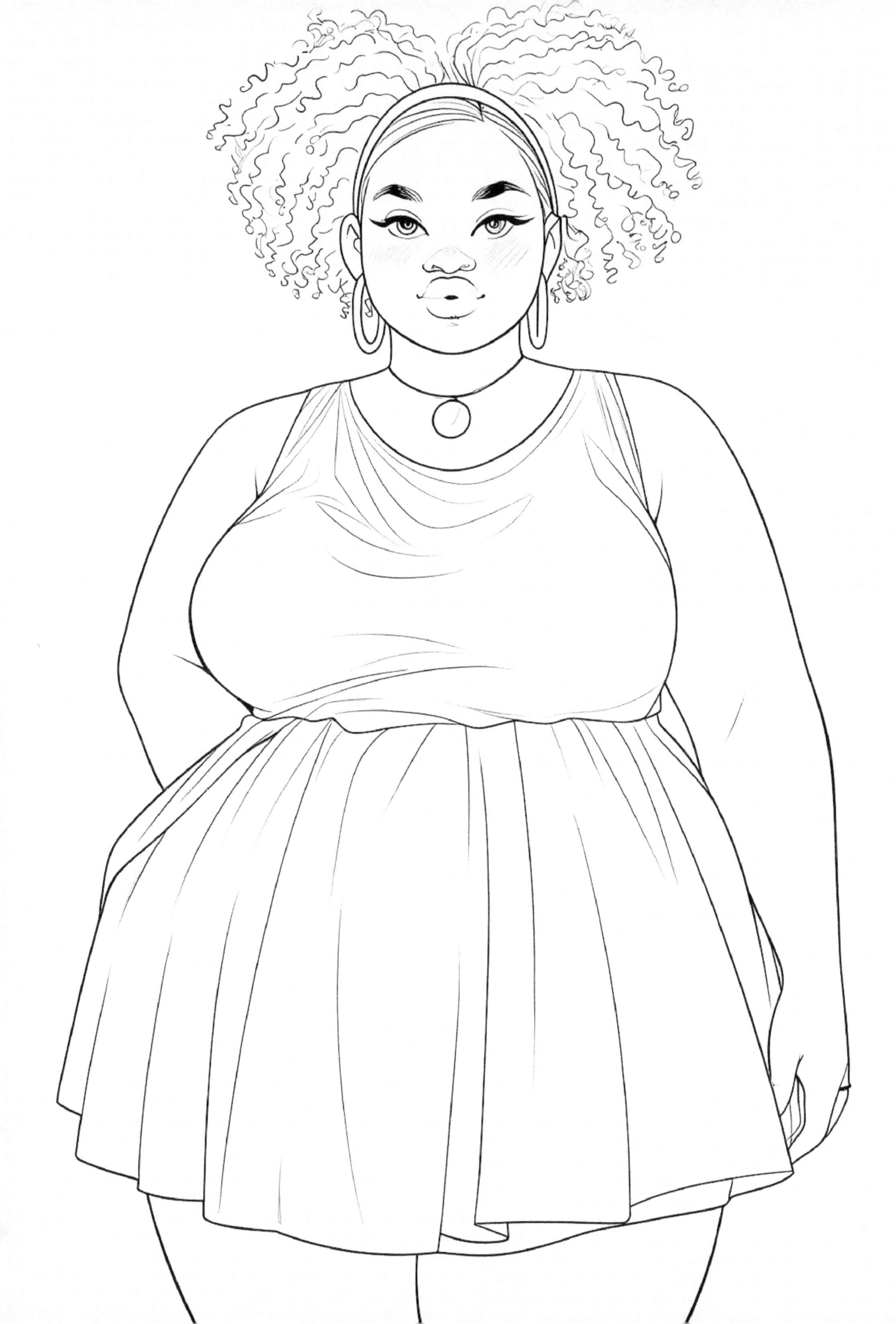

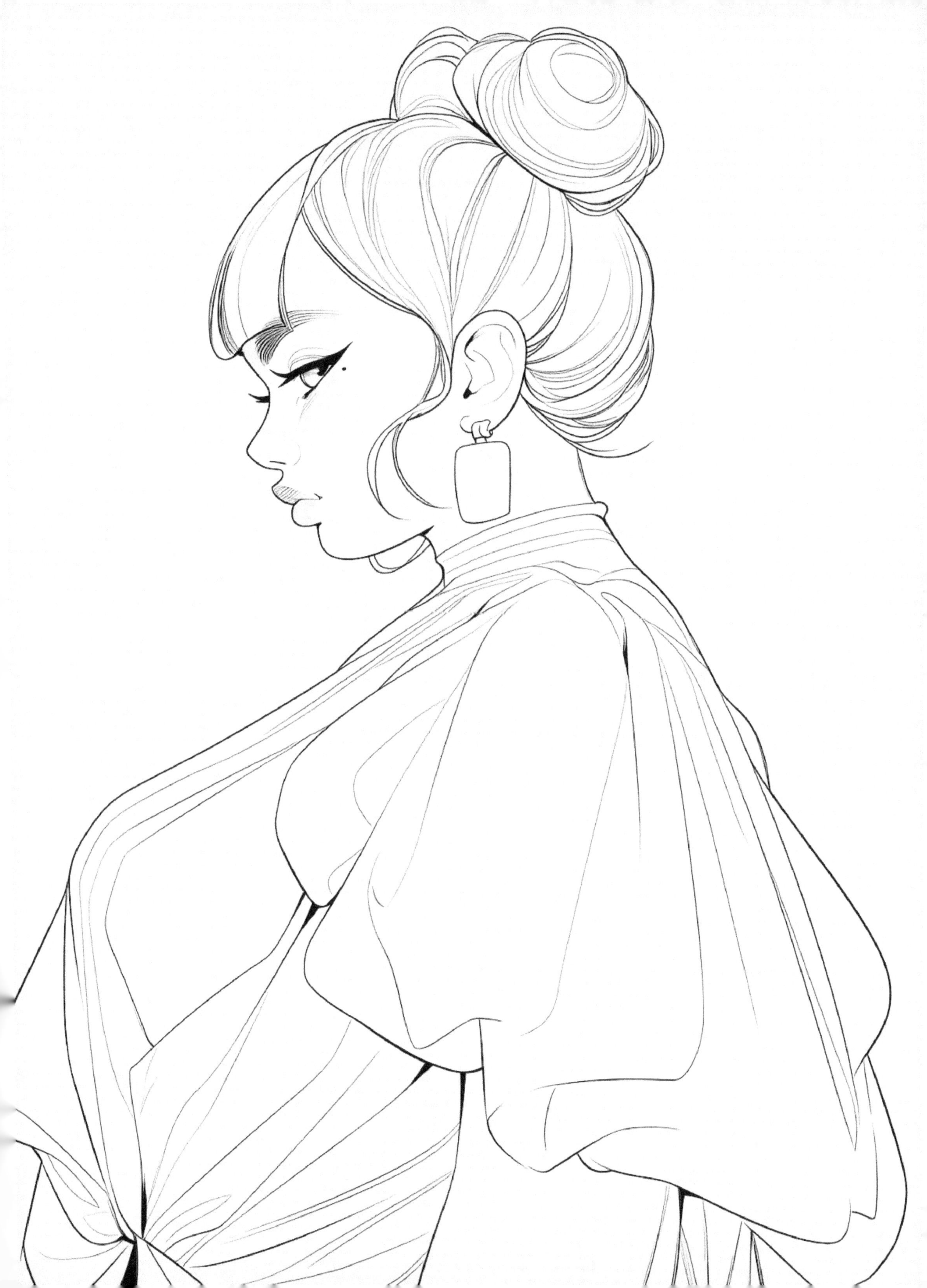

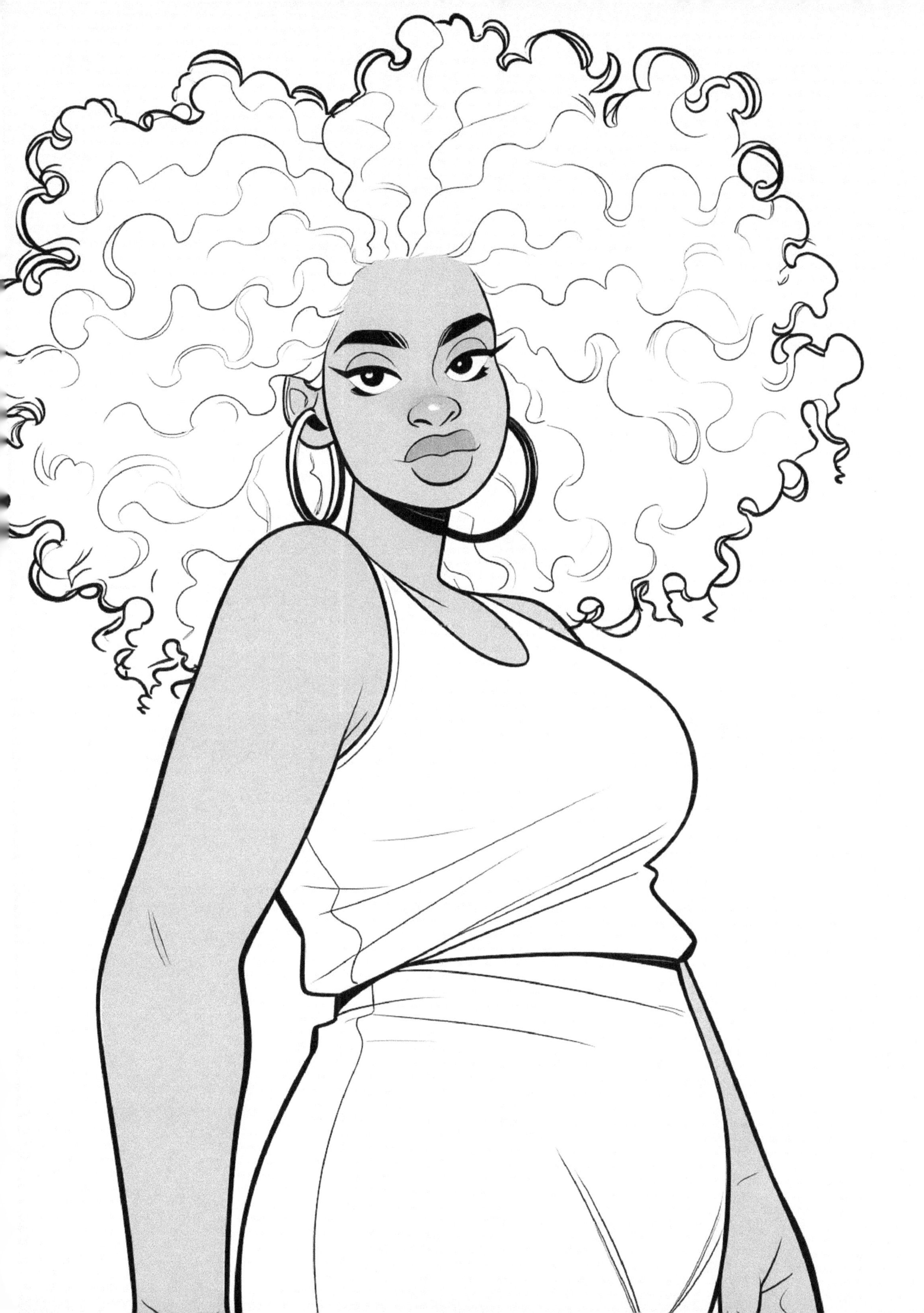

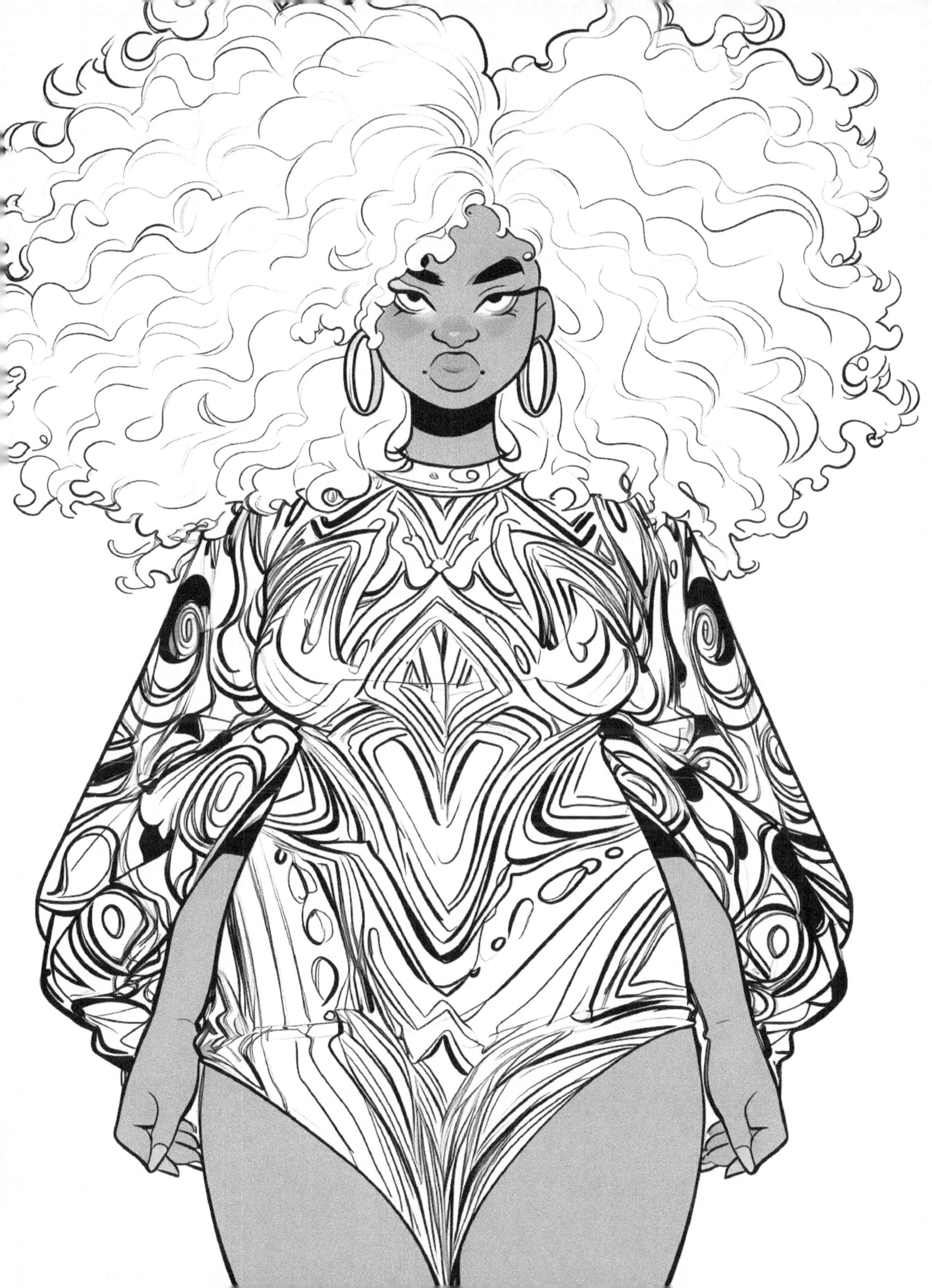

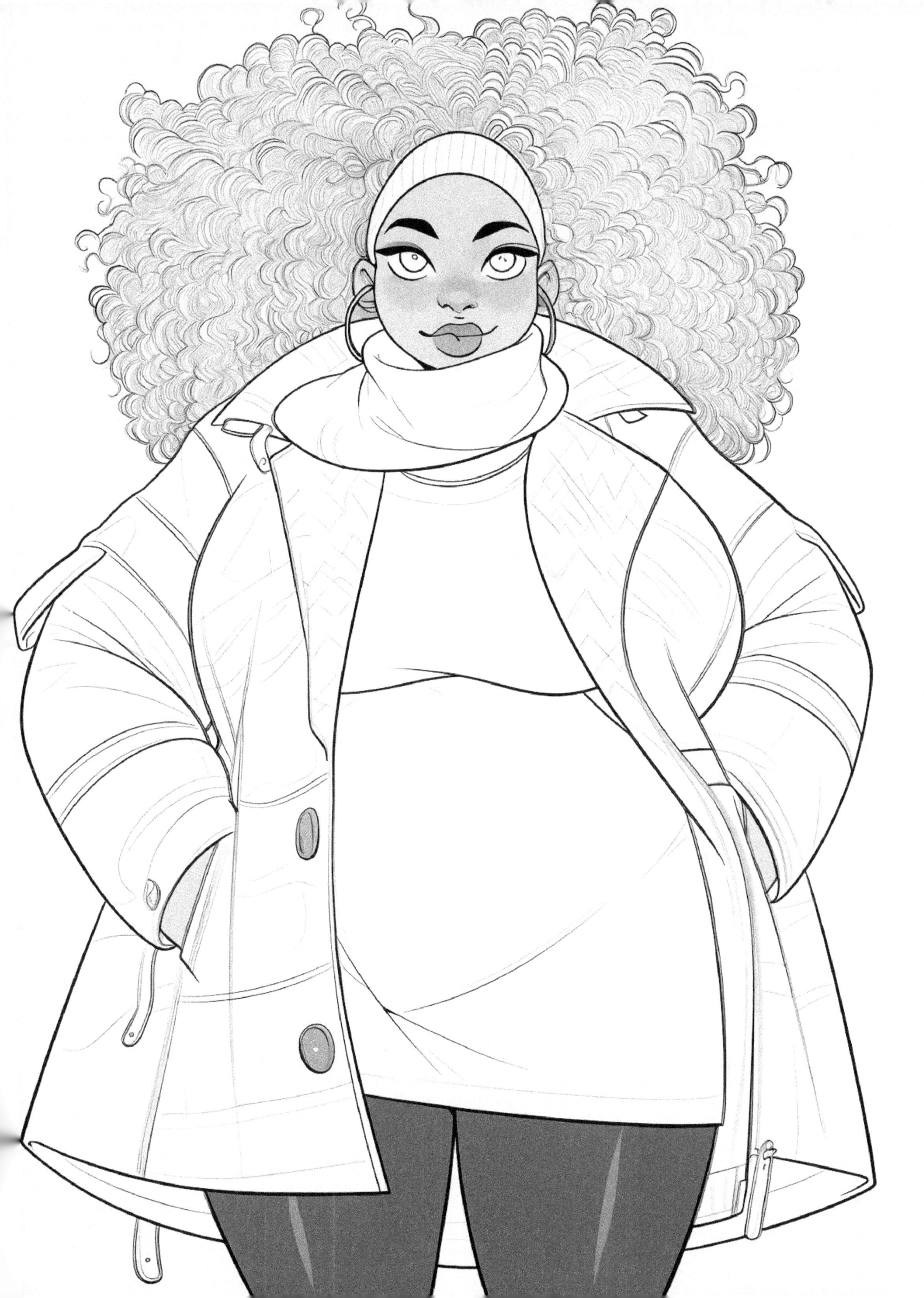

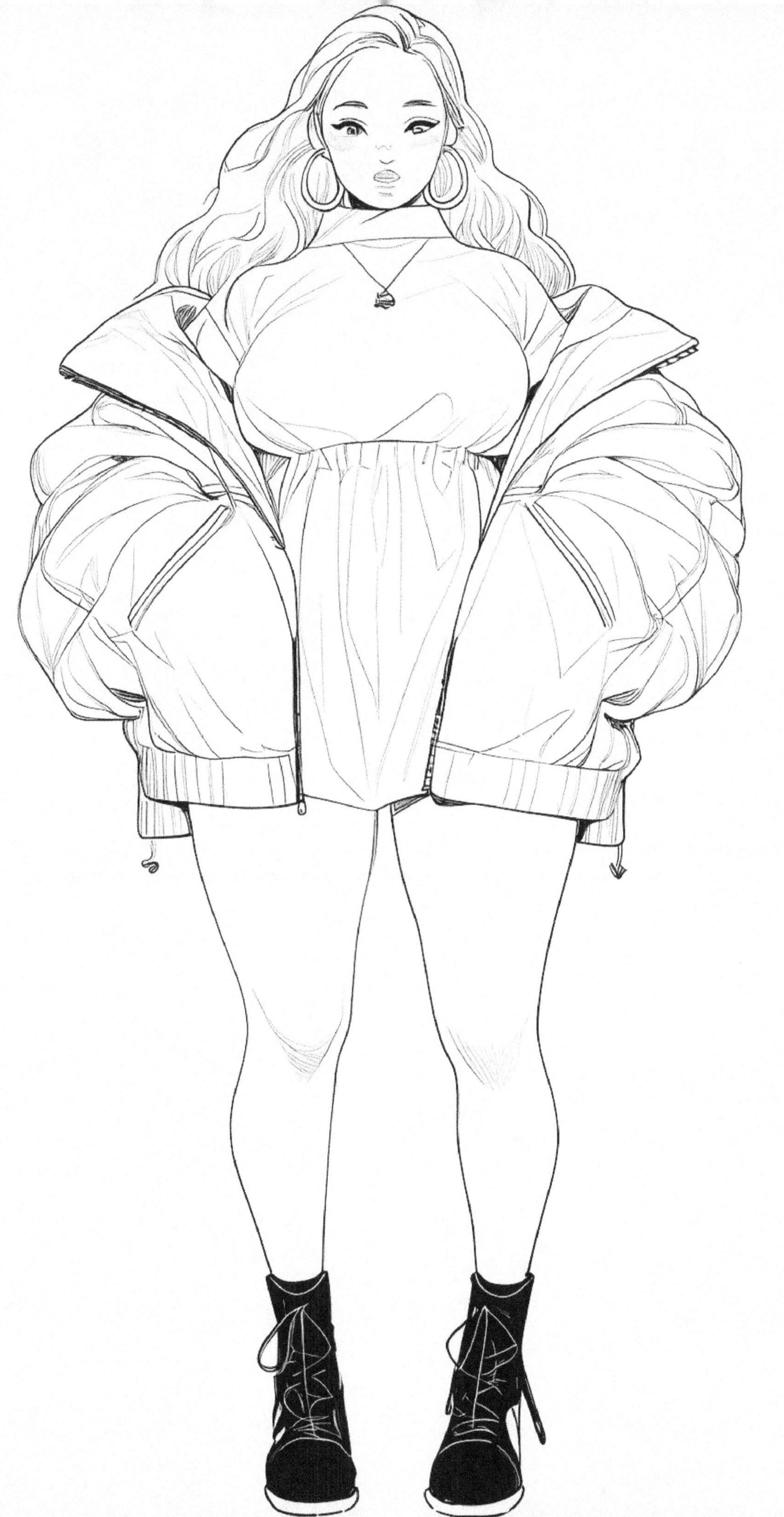

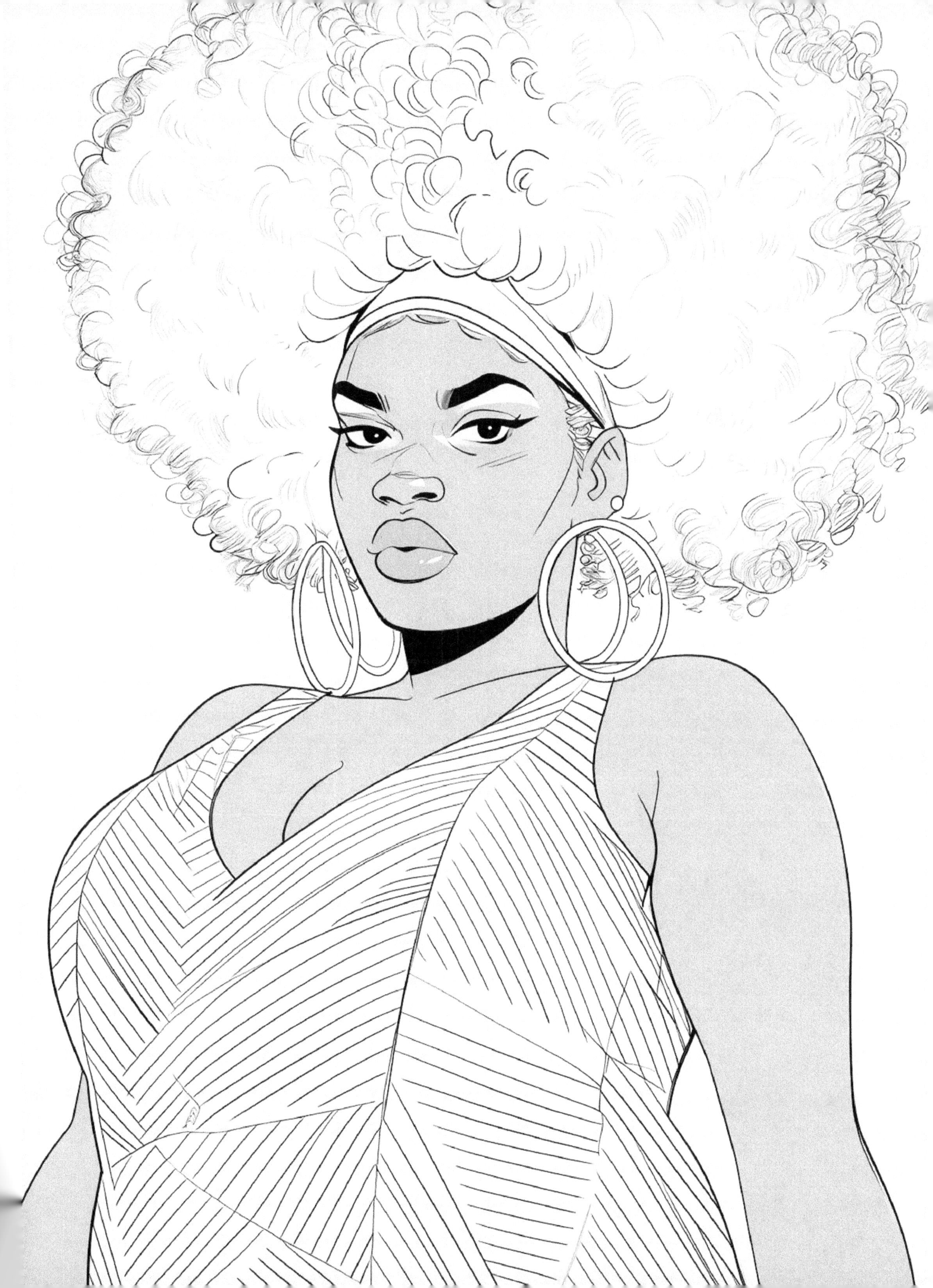

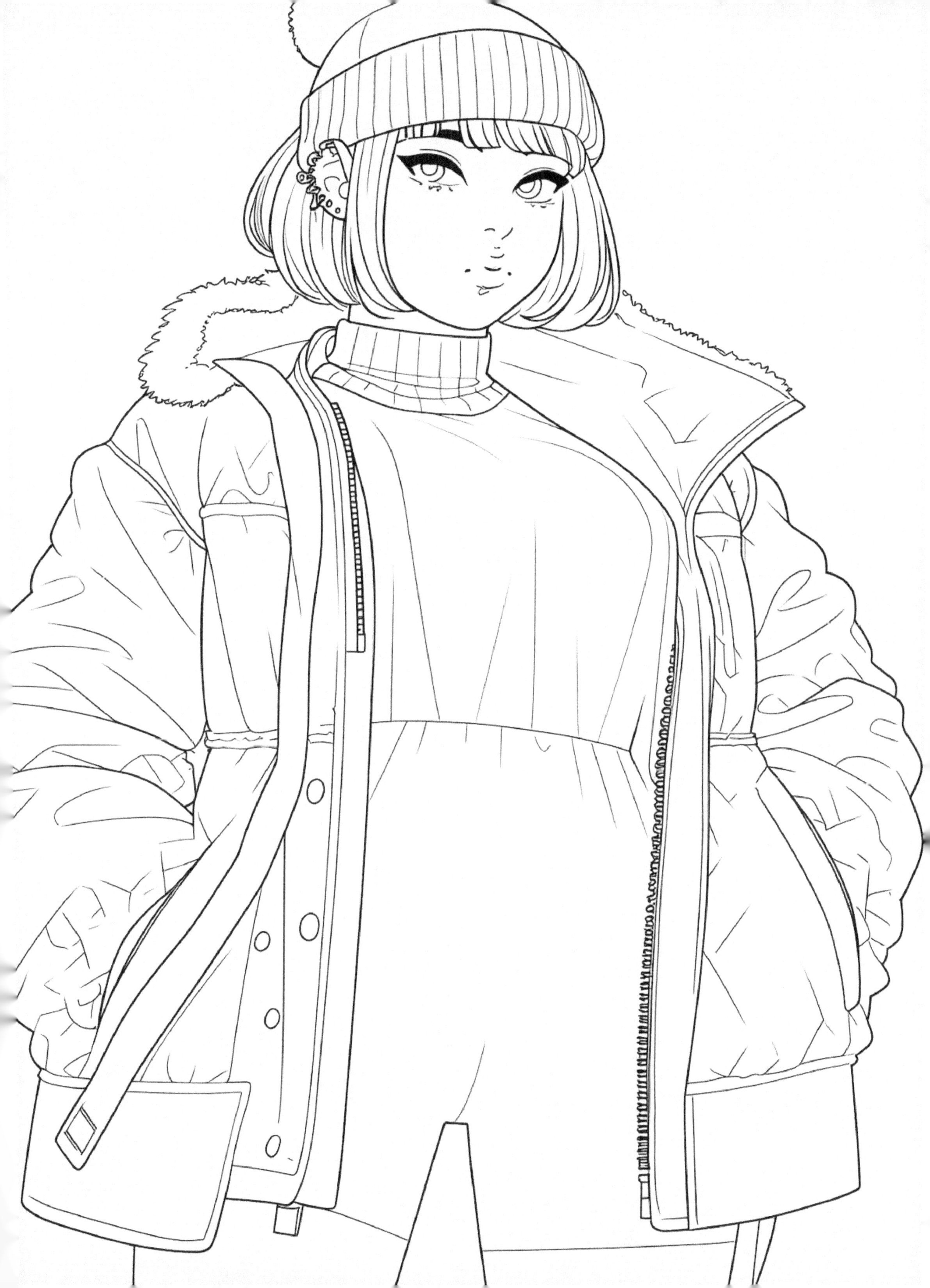

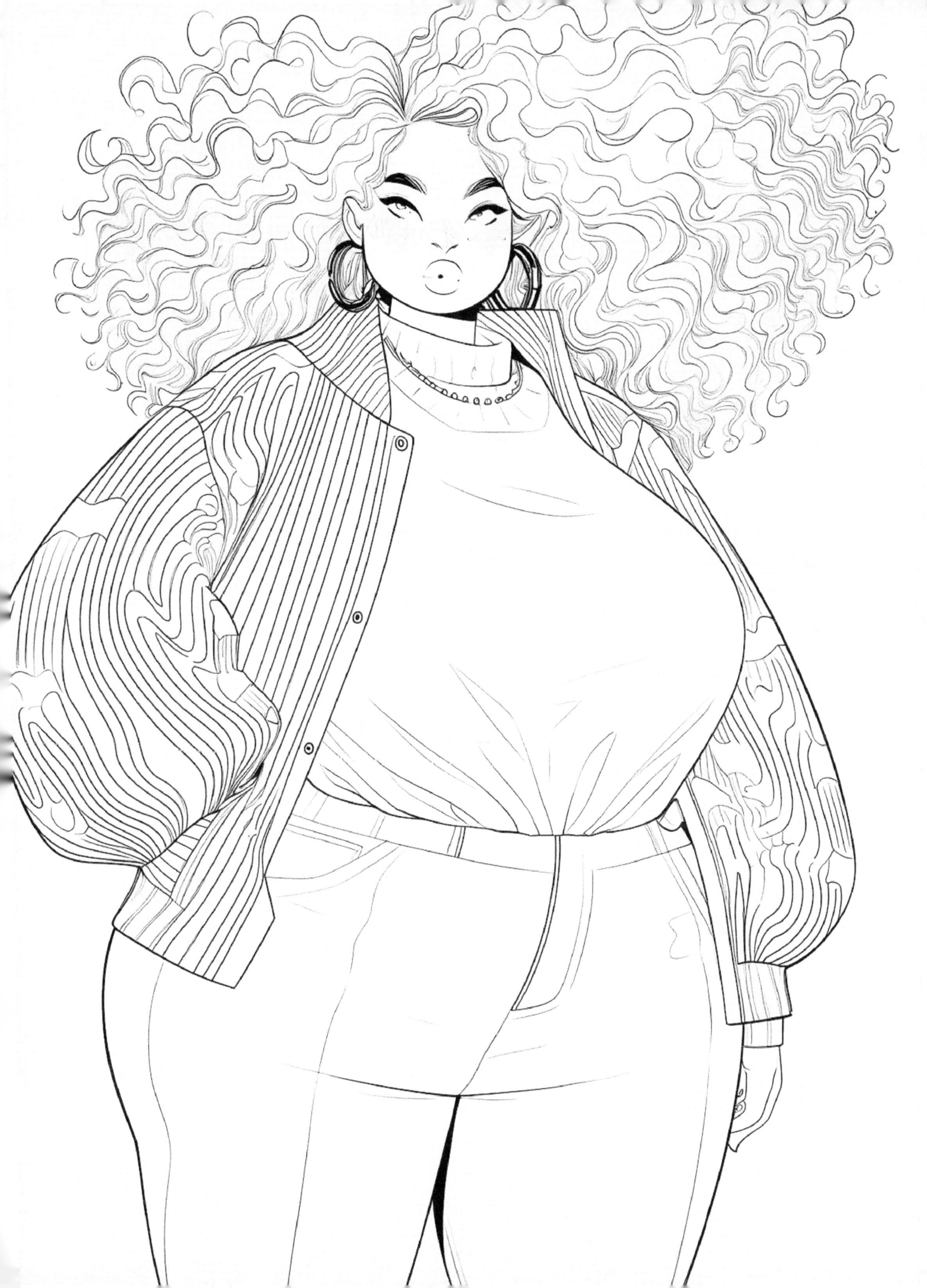

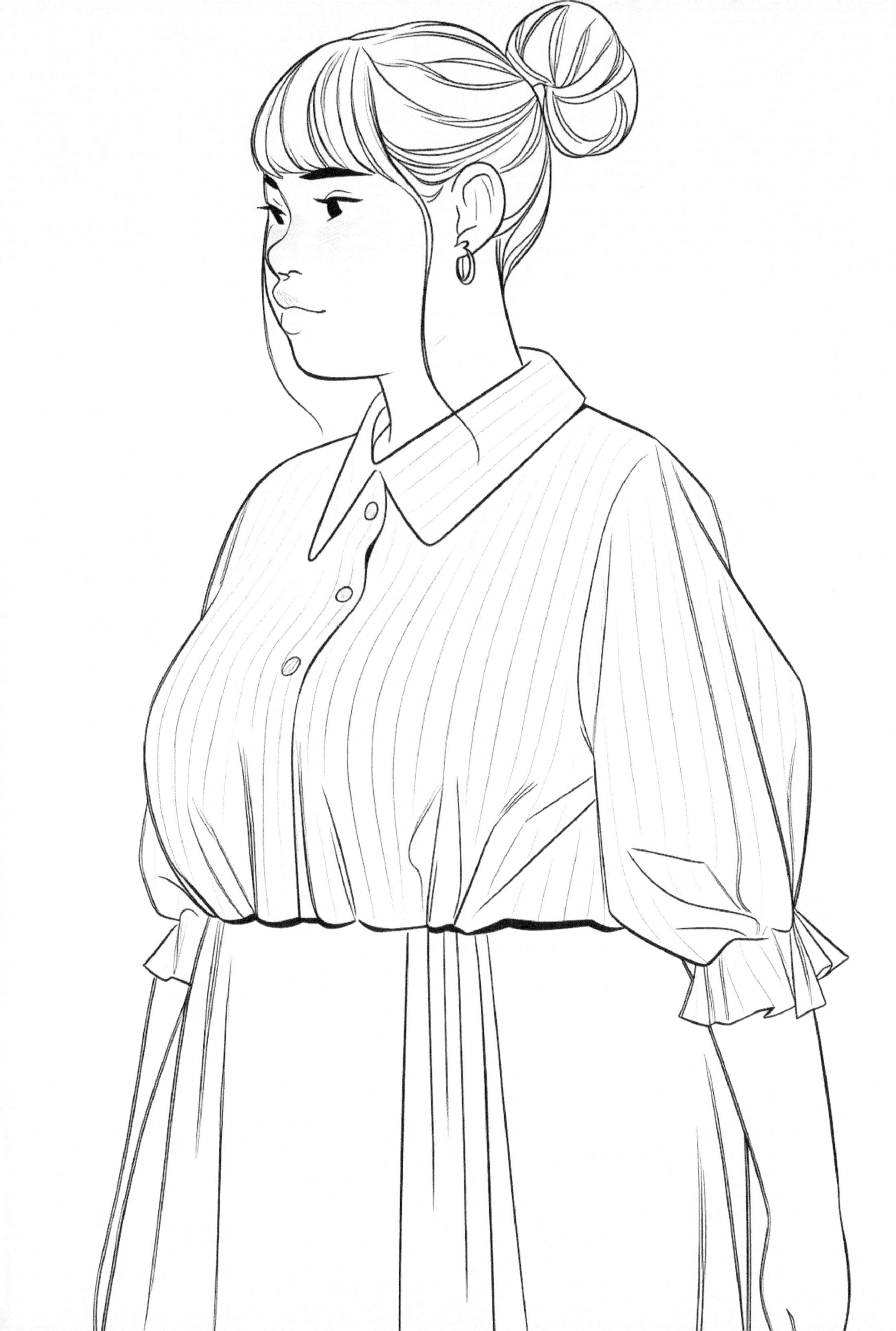

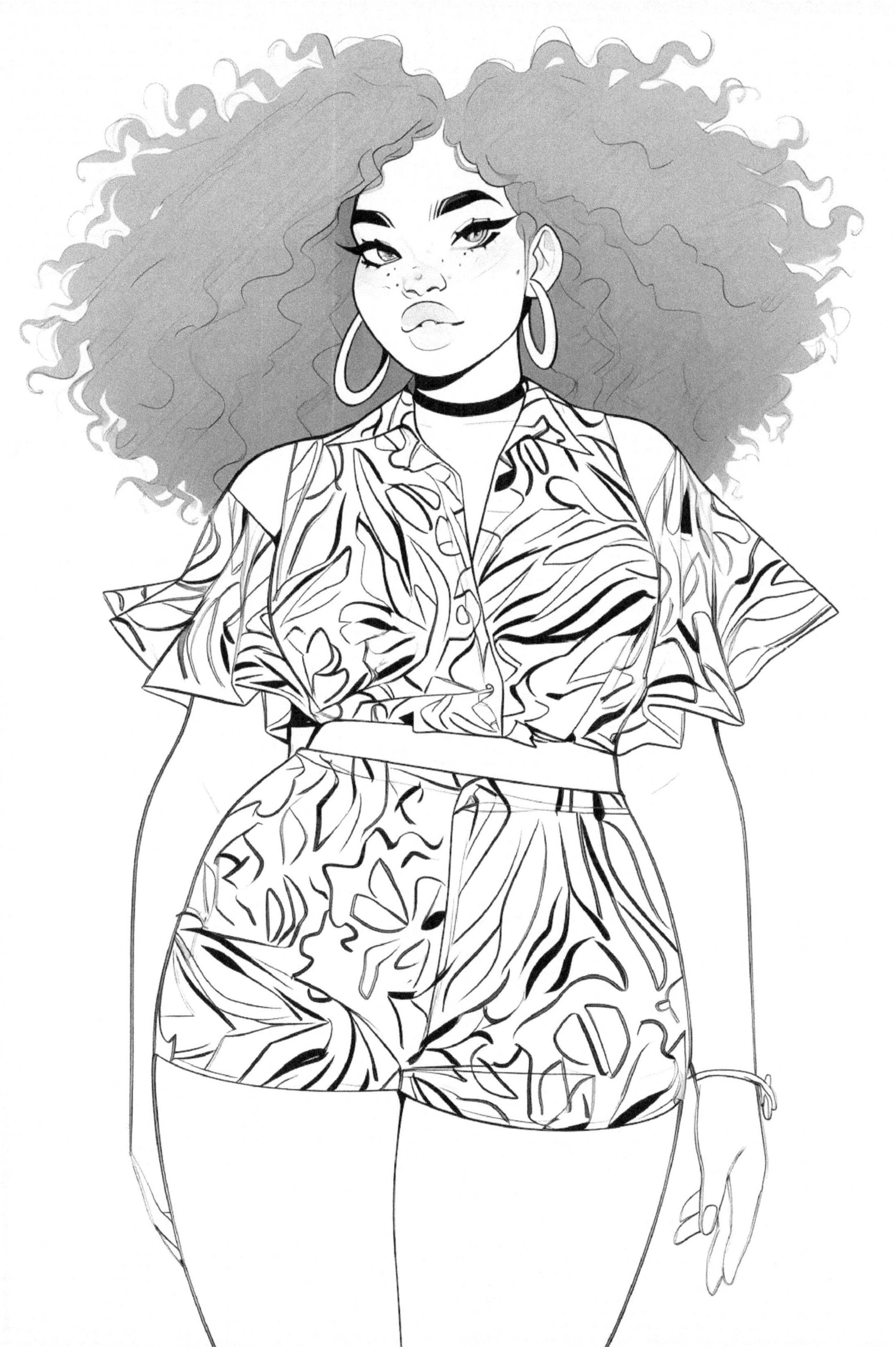

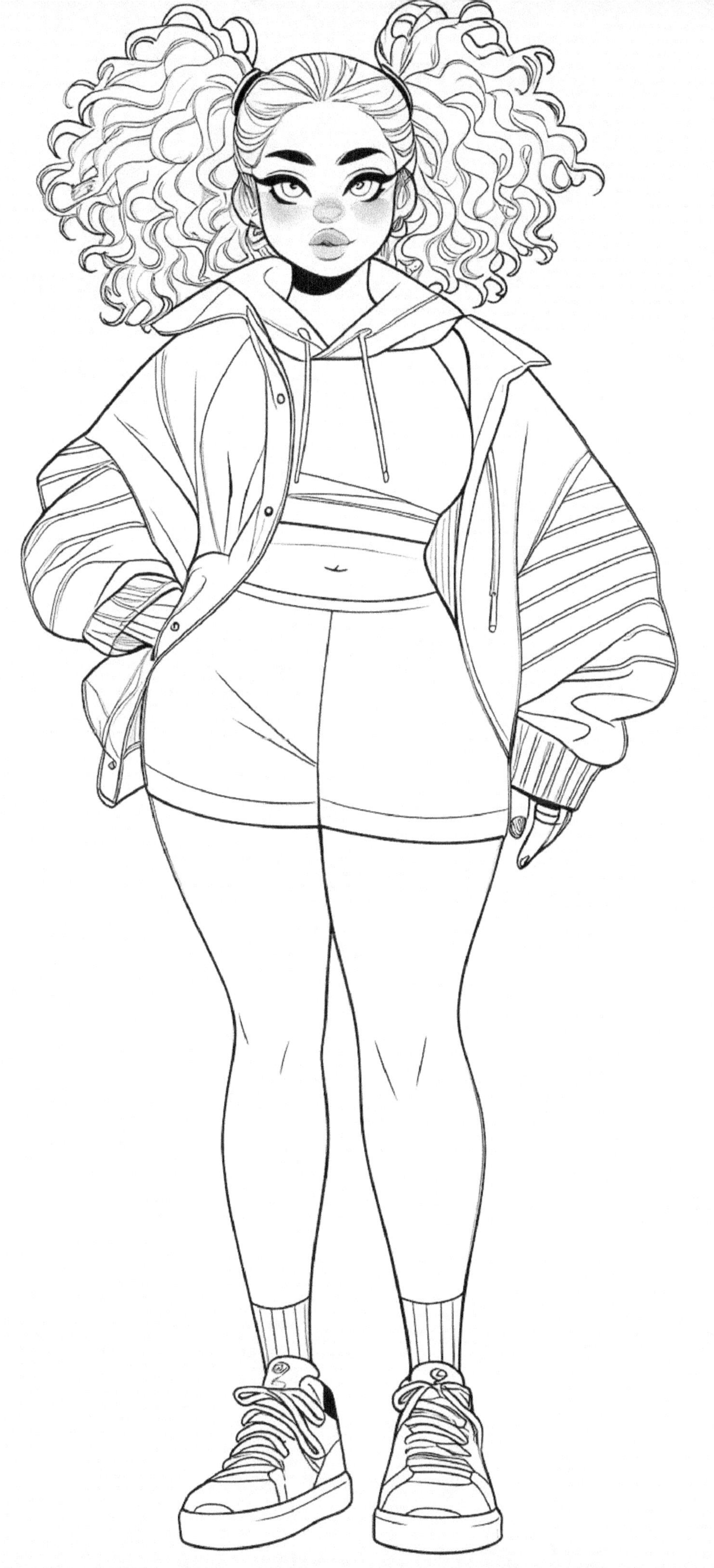

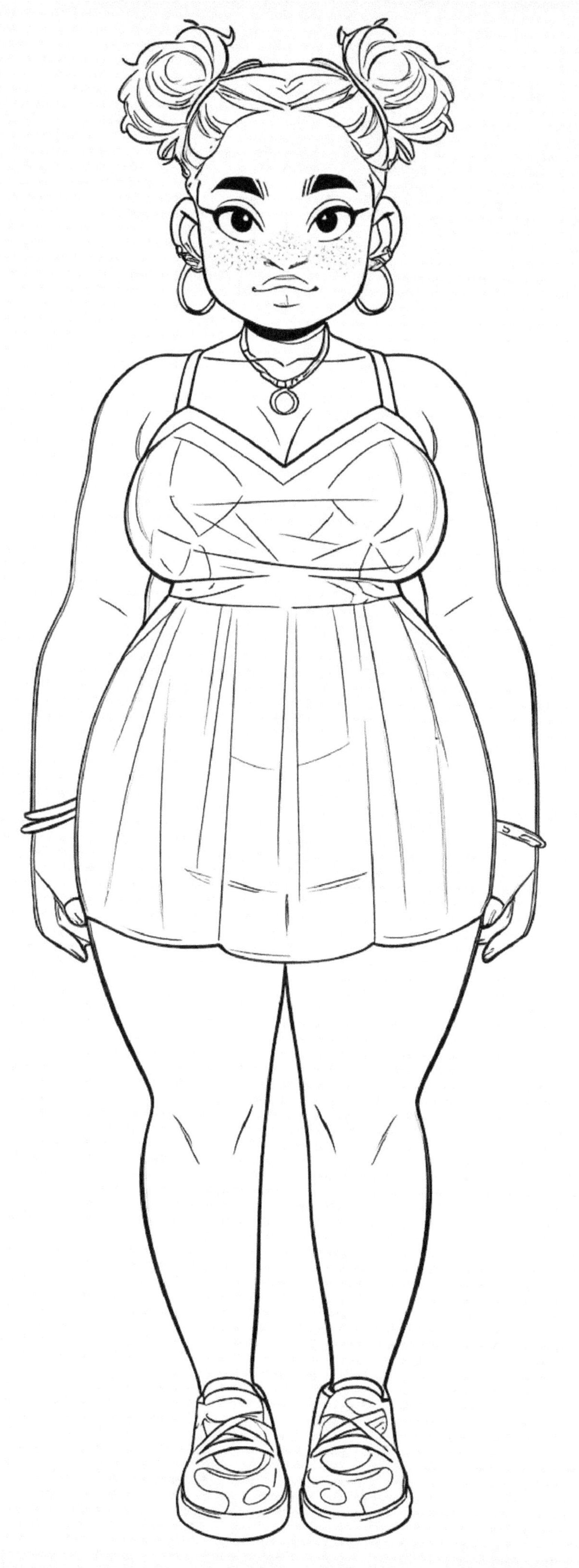

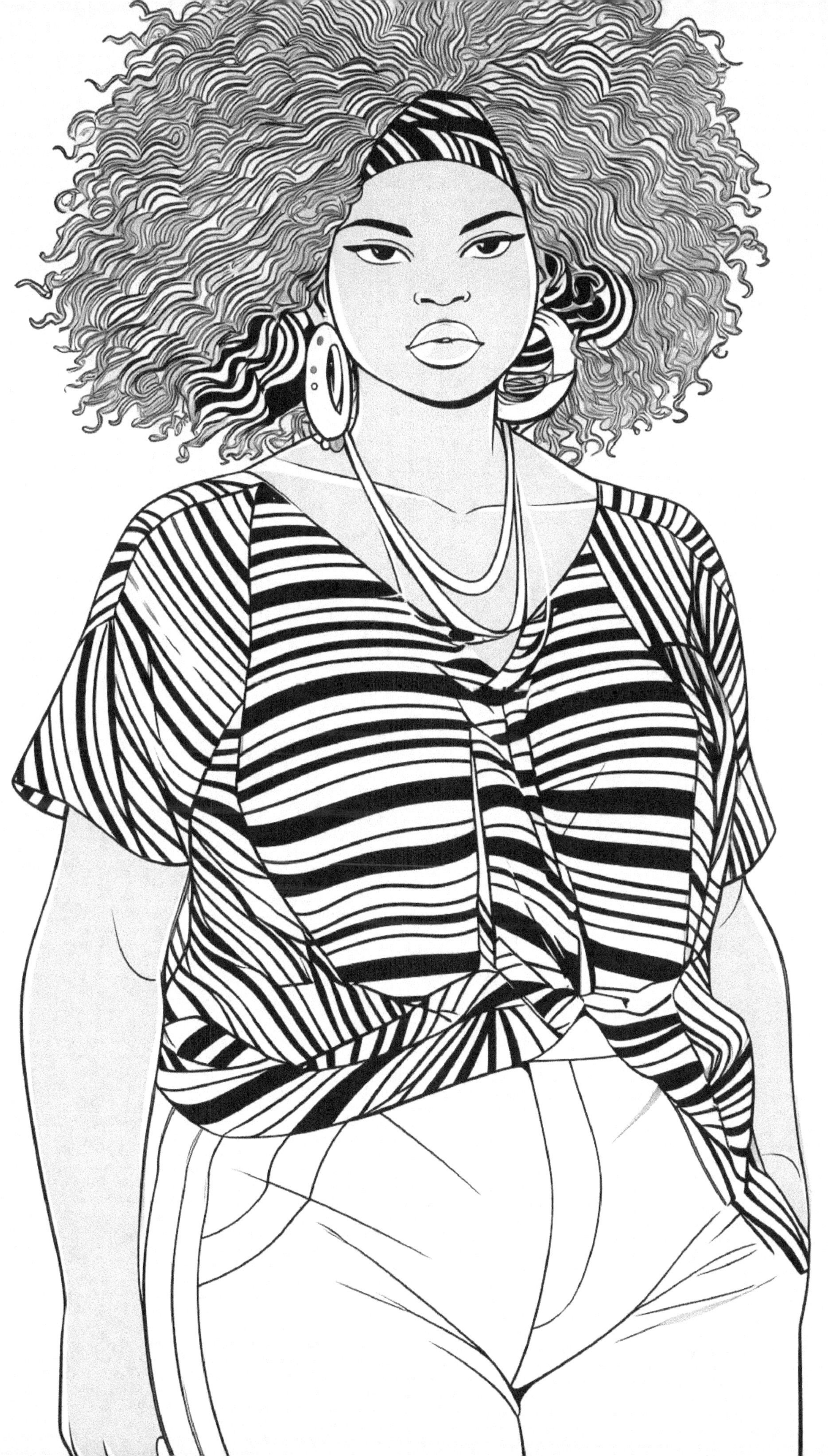

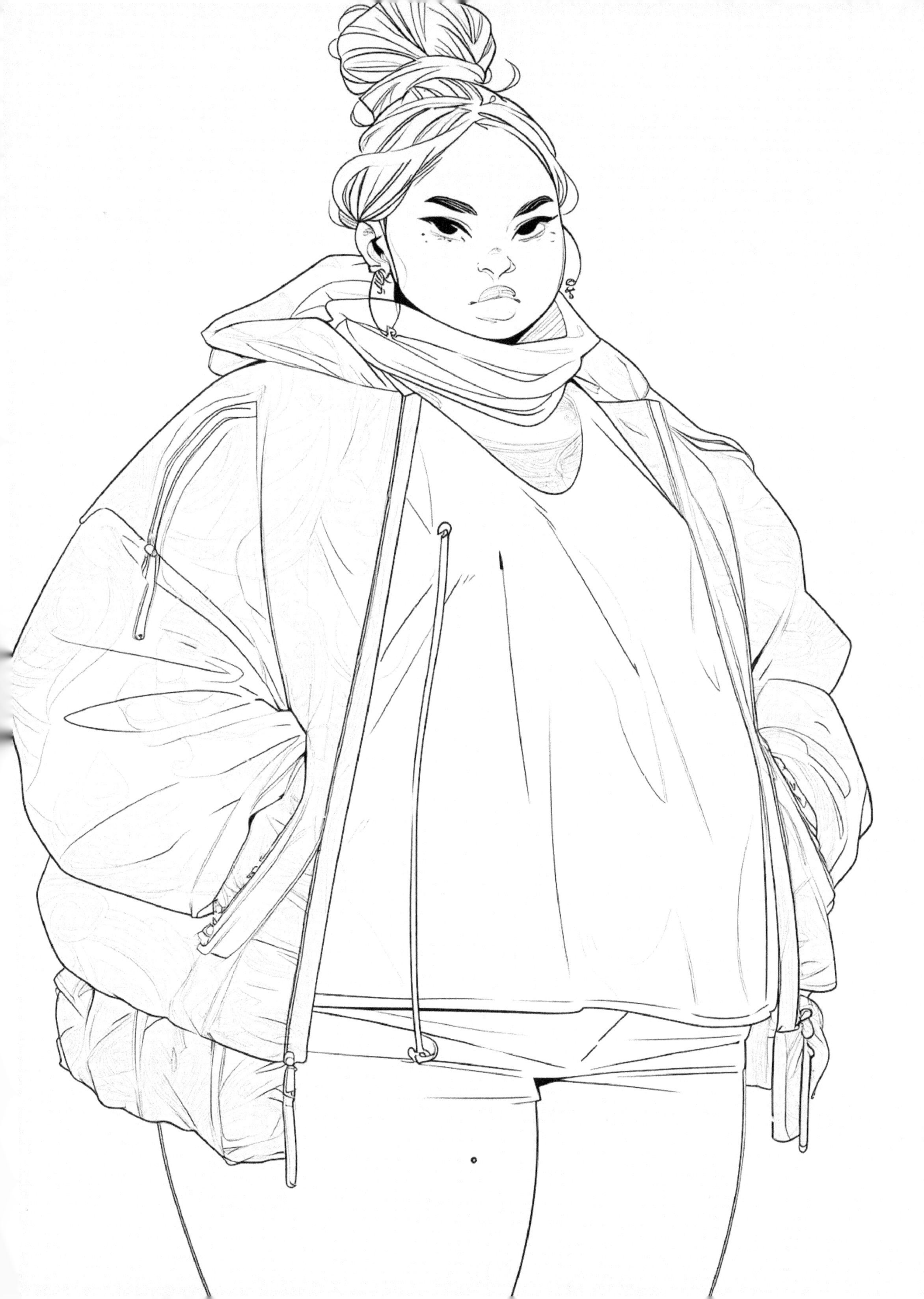

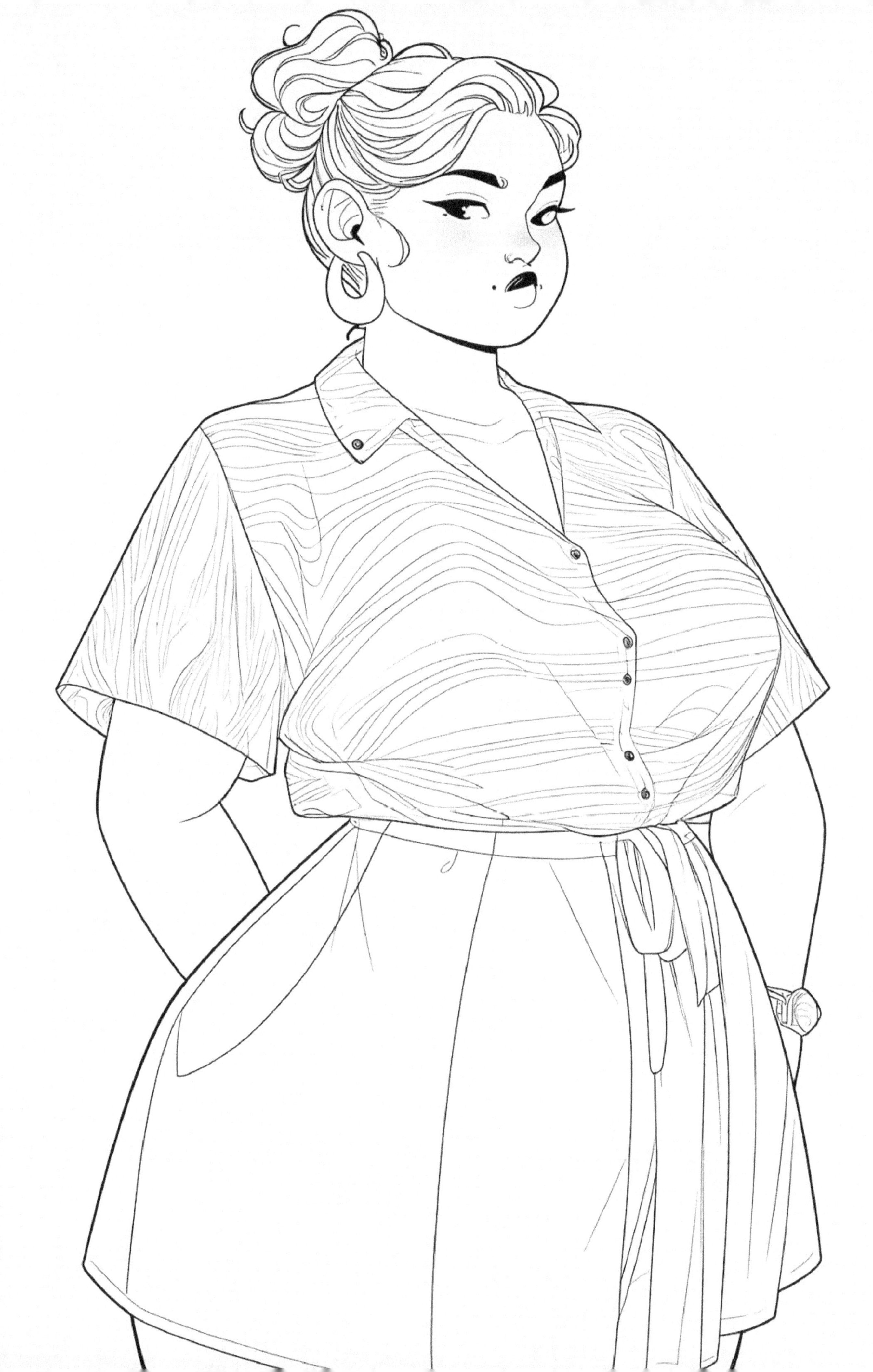

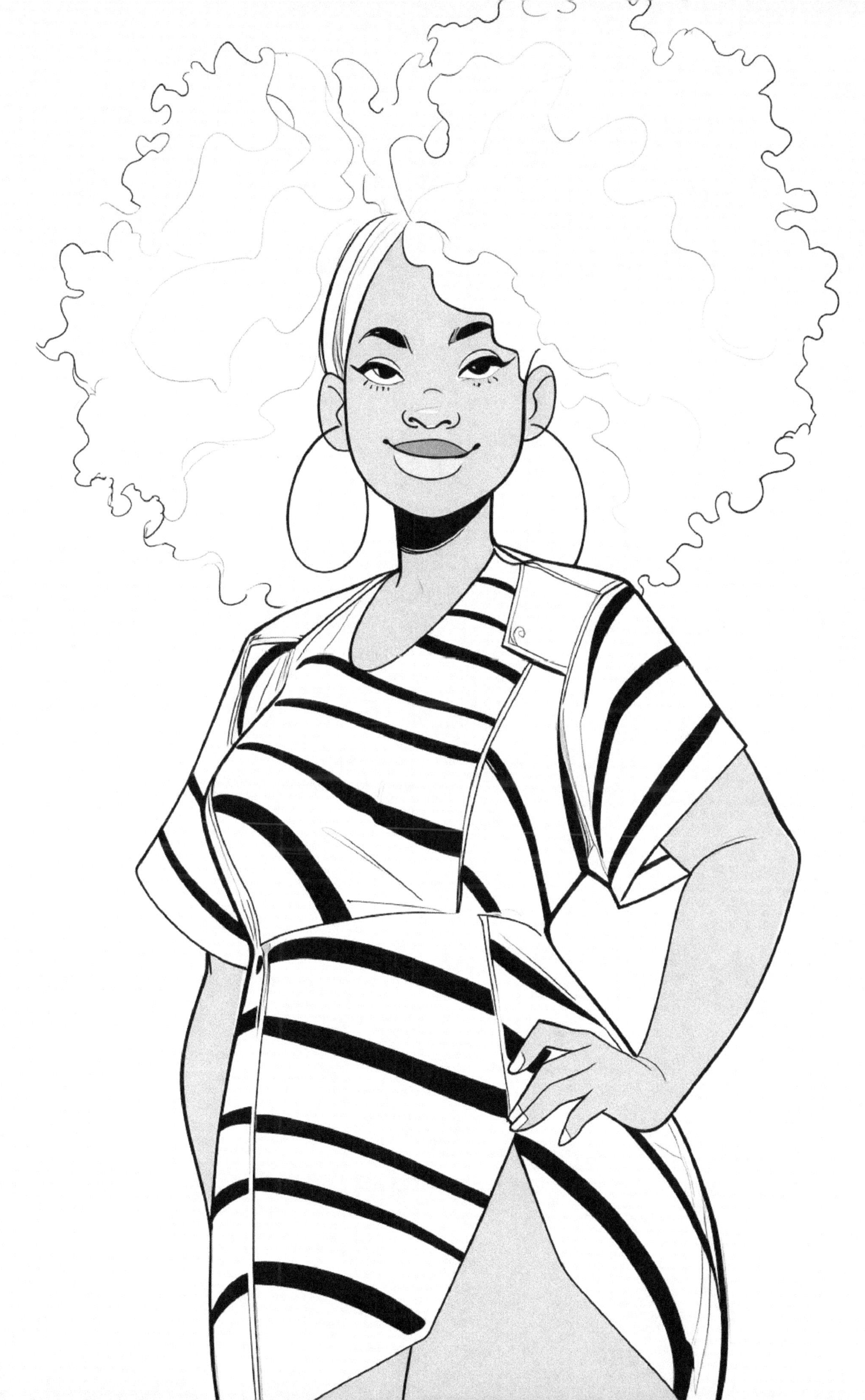

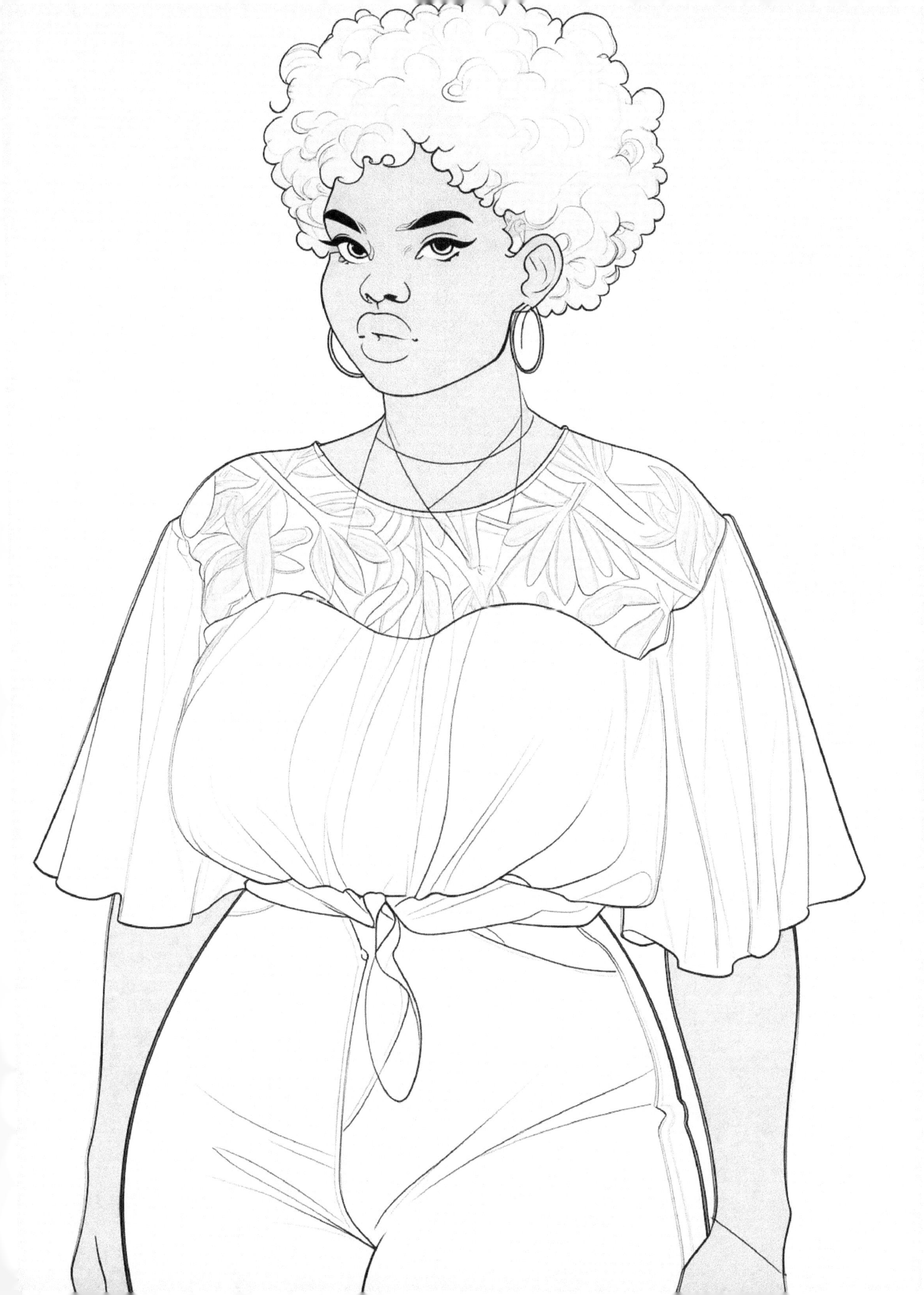

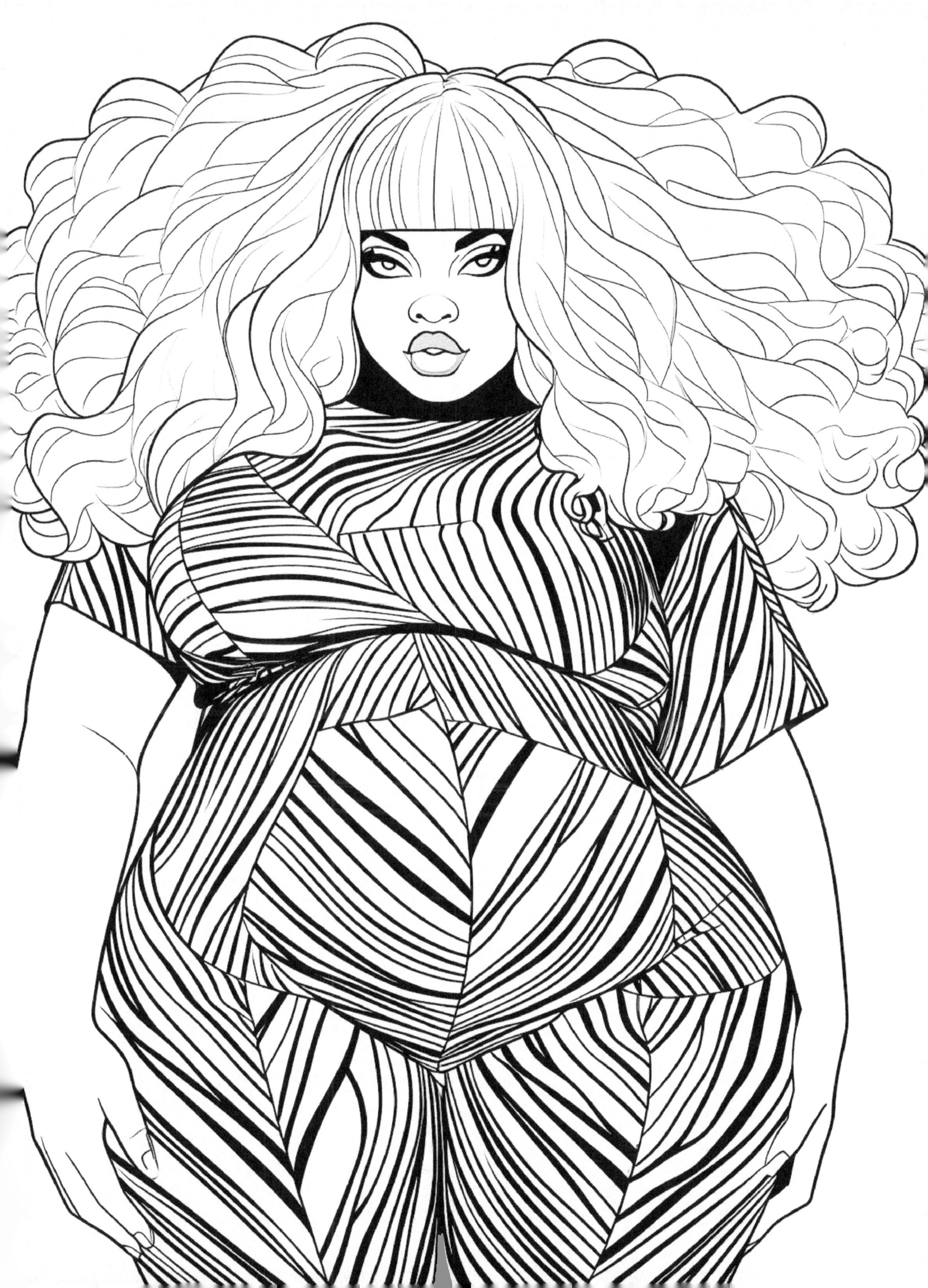

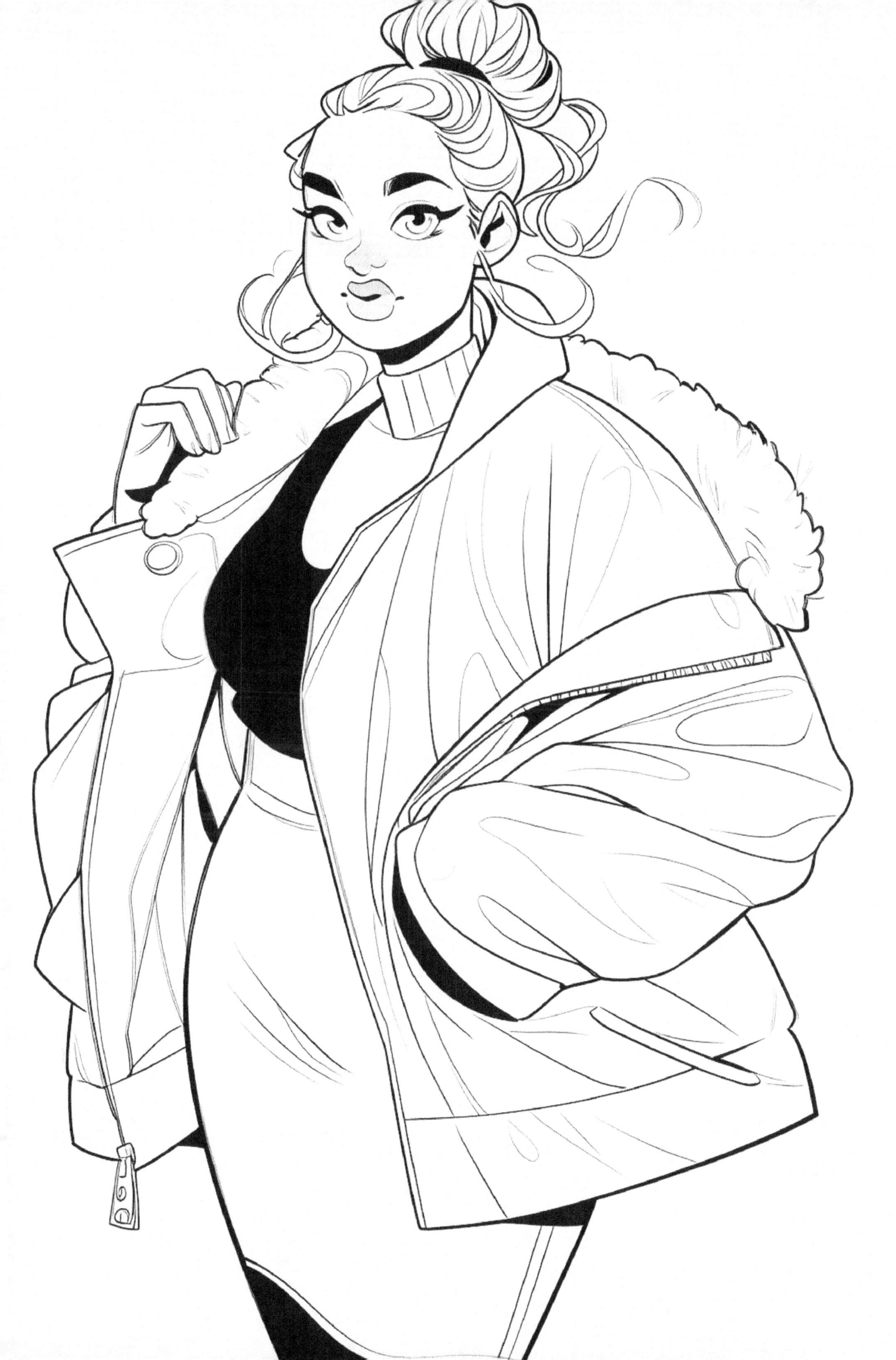

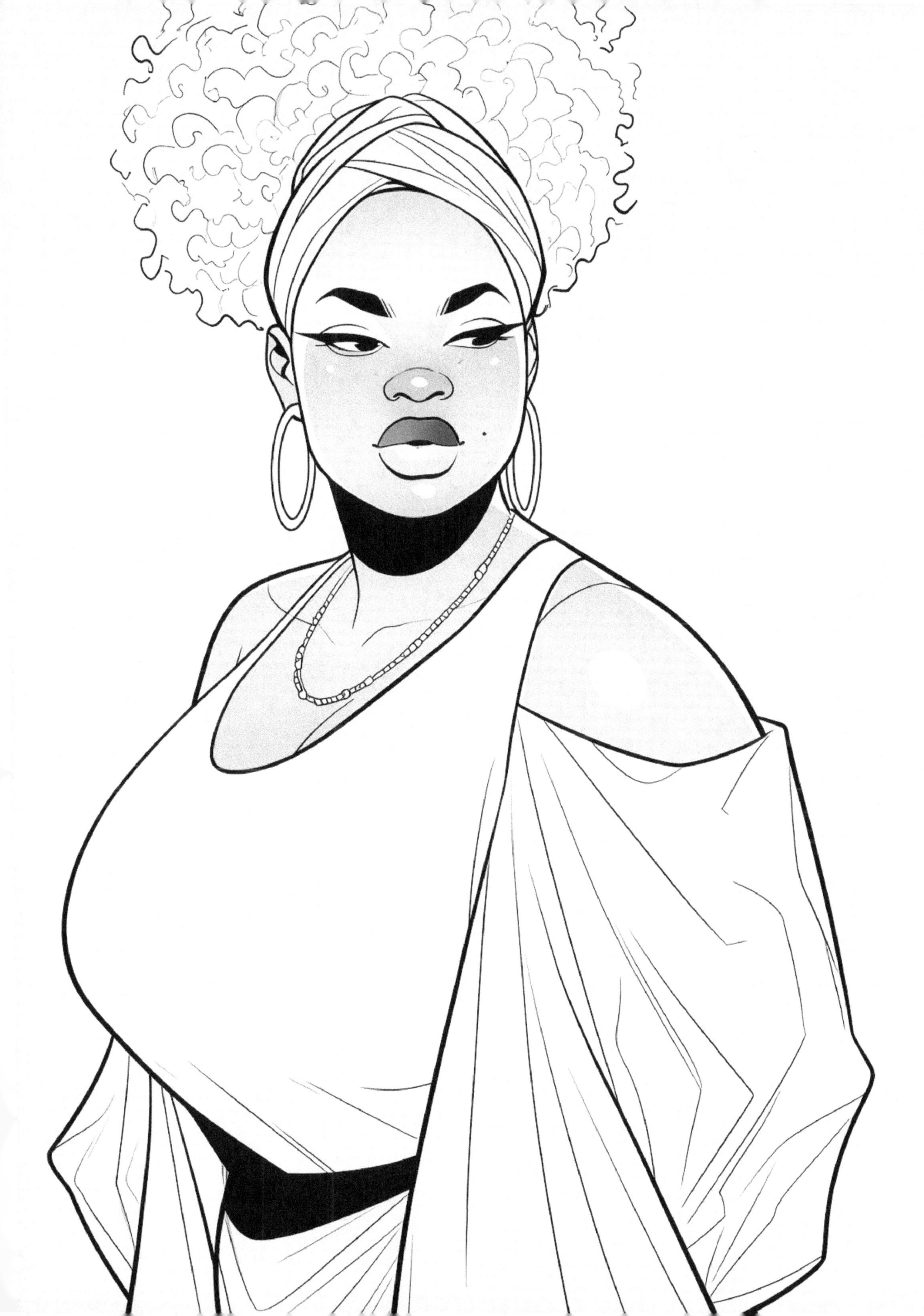

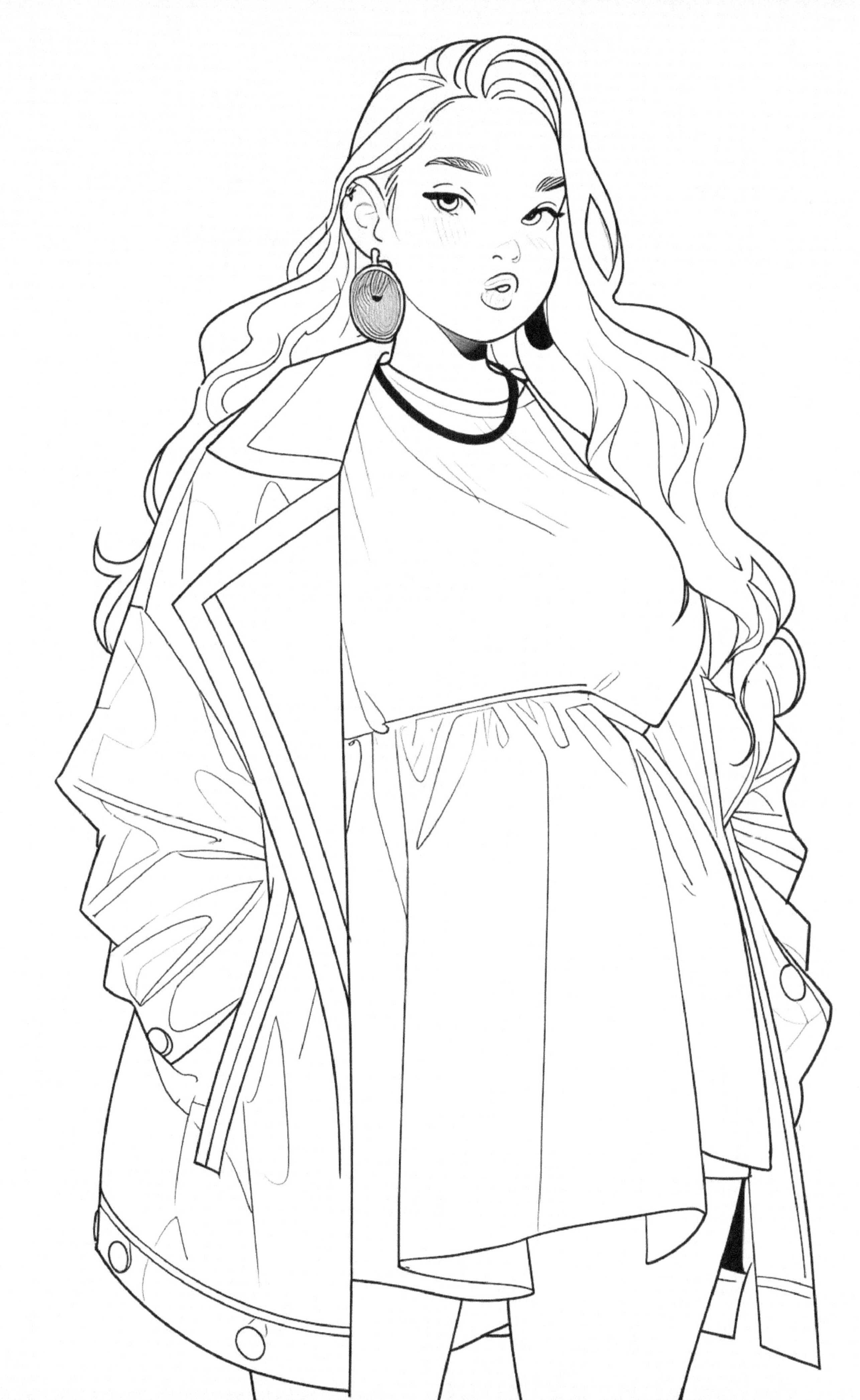

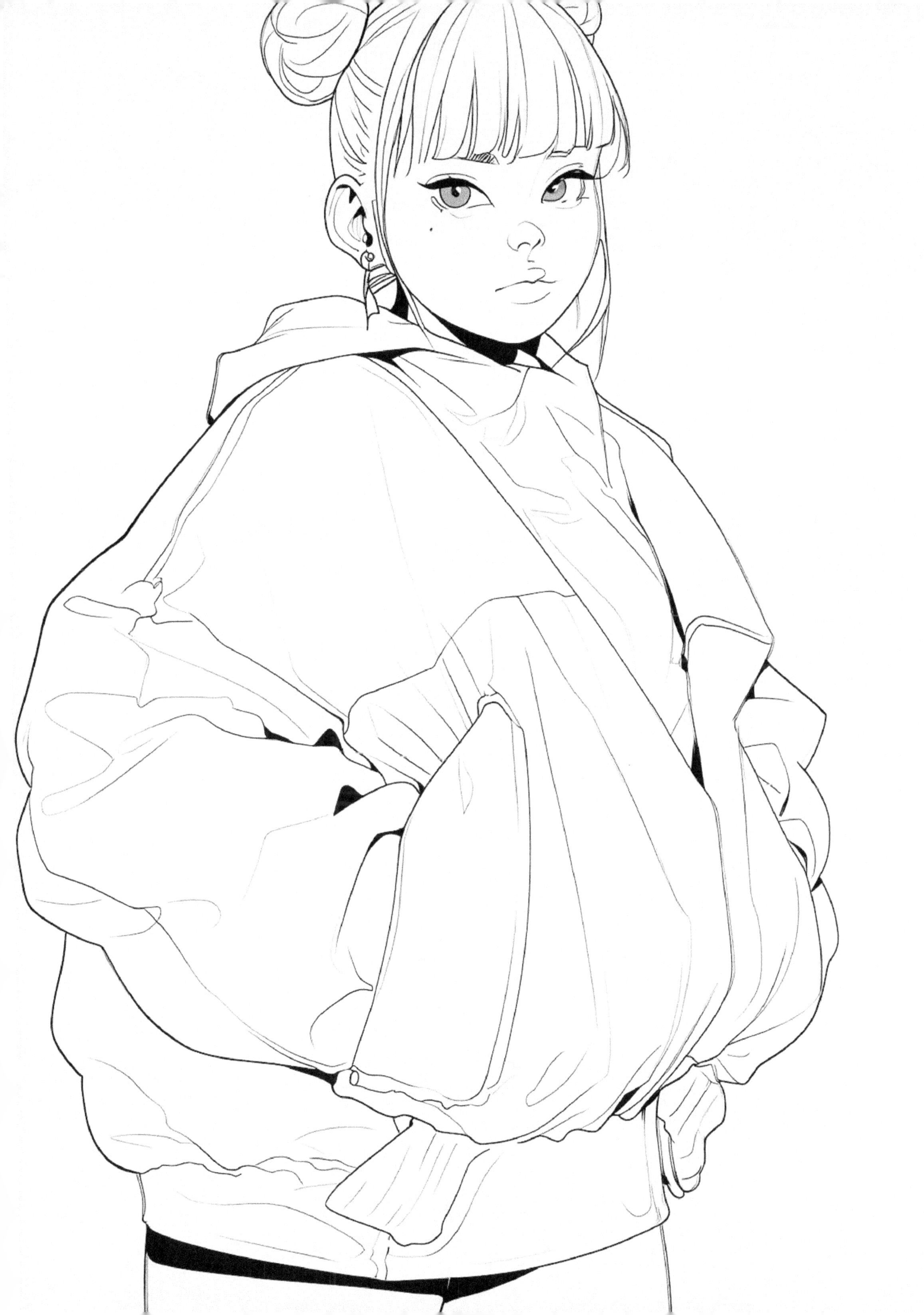